Breathe Better Live Longer

A Practical
Prana Energy Program
for
Wellness & Longevity

Rudra Shivananda

Alight Publications
2015

Breathe Better Live Longer

By Rudra Shivananda

First Edition Published in April 2015

Alight Publications
PO Box 277
Live Oak, CA 95953

http://www.alightbooks.com

Softback ISBN: 978-1-931833-40-0
Ebook ISBN: 978-1-931833-41-7

Printed in the United States of America

For All Those Who
Wish To
Live A Full & Happy
Life

Contents

Introduction

My passion for all aspects of healthy breathing goes back to my early teen years when I was searching for methods to rid myself of the painful effects of high stress. Being an ethnic Indian living in an English colony with the majority of population being Chinese was challenging. The competitive environment to maintain a high scholastic record in a prestigious high school was stressful. I often suffered from headaches and muscular tension that brought on rapid fatigue.

It was natural to look towards the Chinese healing practices that were widely available there and I started to learn about the effects of Chi or life-force energy and how it can alleviate physical imbalances. At fourteen, I was learning to cultivate balance and harmony through movement based Chi exercises. This was tremendously helpful and also led me to seek out some of the sitting-based stillness meditations so that one could find stillness in movement and movement in stillness.

However, I was not satisfied with the effectiveness of these techniques because they did not totally immunize me to stressful situations. Then, I discovered a small book called The Science of Breath by Yogi Ramacharaka and this introduced me to the timeless yogic healing techniques of India.

What I'm sharing with you in this workshop is the essence of the science of breath called pranayama. This yogic science of over four thousand years has been developed for both spiritual and healing purposes. It is a stepping stone to deeper meditation by which one can remove and overcome deep seated psychological problems, as well as the physical maladies that I was initially concerned with.

There is an ancient saying that Breath is Life – we shall be revisiting this wise saying as we proceed during this course. For now, let's consider that when a baby takes its first breath after birth, we consider him or her to be an independent living being. In the

West, we take this moment of first breath as the actual beginning of a life and commemorate it as the birthday. Interestingly enough, a lot can be learned by studying how a healthy baby breathes. As the baby grows up, due to various environmental, karmic and societal influences, he or she develops bad breathing habits that contribute to bad health and shortening of lifespan.

On some level, we are all aware that life ends when breathing stops for more than a few minutes, and yet, we have not paid much attention to the proper maintenance and optimum care of our breath. We take breathing for granted.

There has been a marked improvement in the understanding of proper breathing techniques in the West, due to the continuous influx of Eastern teachers, and the culture of physical health being promoted in the United States and other affluent societies for the last thirty years. Unfortunately, there has been a concomitant decrease in the healthy breathing habits of the masses in developing countries, such as India itself, due to the priority given to Western education and application of outdated nineteenth century beliefs. Today, even in the land of Yoga and enlightened sages, school children are taught the unhealthy habit of inhaling, while pulling in the abdomen, without using the diaphragm, restricting the expansion of the lungs and decreasing the amount of air that can reach the body's organs.

Most people still breathe with only about a third of their lung capacity. By learning how to breathe properly to strengthen and extend the respiratory capacity can give a tremendous healing boost to the vital organs which have been habitually starved for oxygen and bathed in carbon dioxide waste. Therefore the first part of the book focuses on developing Breath Awareness, and to learning the practice of the **Complete Breath**, also called the Full Yogic Breath. By regular breathing in a deeper and fuller manner, the quality of one's life will greatly improve. It has been observed that even long-term physiological problems have been healed by the regular practice of the Complete Breath.

Also in the first part of the book we will examine the causes of stress and it's debilitating efffects on physical and emotional health. We will then learn the life-saving de-stressing breath called the **Calming Breath**.

In the second part, I will introduce the concept of the vital energy called Prana or Chi which is responsible for the well-ness of the body, mind and emotions. We will then bring into our lives the energising techniques called the **Energy Balance** and and **Moving Energy Booster**.

In the third part, we delve deeper into the dynamics of how breath can further increase well-ness and longevity. We will examine the subtle anatomy of our physiology and learn about the heating and cooling energies in the body, about the five functional pranas and the five elemental categories . It is the imbalances in the subtle forces that contribute to the decay and disease of the physical body. Their imblance also contribute to emotional issues such as depression which reduces the will to life. We will learn to balance these subtle energies and forces within us with the **Sun-Moon Breath**, the **Five-Prana Breath** and the **Five-Elements** Breath.

I've been a student and teacher of breathing for over forty years and have spent thousands of hours working with the techniques in this course. They have contributed tremendously to my well-being and that of many of my students. Although, I've relied on the teachings of the great Masters that have come before us and my own experiential contributions, it should be emphasized that there is a lot of positive scientific research that backs up the effectiveness of breath work in dealing with many common but difficult psychological and physical problems. There are hundreds of scientific studies that can be accessed on the web concerning the use of breathing techniques as treatment for problems such as depression, anxiety, asthma, high blood pressure and gastro-intestinal maladies.

In this course, I've put together a well-ness program that will be helpful for preventing many health problems among young people and to heal many of the problems attacking older people like myself. The techniques in this program were chosen because they will show rapid if not immediate results with the investment of a short duration of practice. Ten to fifteen minutes per day for healthy maintenance and half an hour for treatment purposes should be sufficient. Everyone who practices these techniques find their energy level and mental acuity noticeably boosted in a day or two. This is important because it motivates them to consciously make an effort to regularly practice, which in turn produces more positive results.

You will also find much of the foundational knowledge that will help you understand better how this program of better breathing will contribute to your well-being and longevity.

Part 1

*The Physical Body
&
Breath Awareness*

Breathing is both a conditioned behavior, and a voluntary action - it is a dynamic, multifaceted, vital function of the body combining physiology and psychology. Physiologically, breathing occurs automatically based upon needs of the body and is directly related to its metabolism. The word metabolic is used to describe a biochemical process in the body—the buildup of some substances and the breakdown of others. On a cellular level, breathing brings about the exchange of oxygen and carbon dioxide that has built up in the blood. You know that when you run fast or when you are suffering from a high fever, your body needs more oxygen to be pumped quickly. Our heart rate and our breathing rate are linked for this reason - they both speed up and slow down at the same time – naturally occurring in the background without any conscious effort on our part. Even though we don't know the science behind it all, we can have experienced the effect.

Our psychology – perception and emotions, can also influence our breath. We have individual and particular emotional temperaments that are determined by our genes, our family environment, and our

> *Science shows that your health is directly related to how you breathe.*

life experiences. These variables cause our breathing to change in rate, depth, and quality in reaction to emotions. Thinking about something in the past that upsets us, or something in the future that excites can increase the breathing rate and disturb its pattern. Similarly, if we are currently experiencing something pleasant or unpleasant, our breath will change.

Over time, repeated reactions to inner and outer conditions become ingrained like any practice or habit. We unconsciously associate breathing patterns with stimuli, and therefore breathing patterns are reinforced and generalized showing that breathing is also a conditioned behavior, a habitual response. The more often certain emotions are associated with certain experiences, the more breathing will shift and settle into a pattern, which may not always be healthy. For example, as a child, you may have a parent who was critical of your behavior in certain situations and this may have caused you to hold your breath in those situations and tense your whole body. After repeatedly experiencing this, you may feel anxious, your respiratory rate may increase, and you may hold extra tension in your muscles. In later life, this pattern of holding the breath may lead to asthmatic behavior – it has become automatic and generalized to being in a stressful situation.

A unique characteristic of the breath is that it can be under voluntary control - we can hold our breath, or breathe faster, or breathe slower, at any time, by choice. It is the only visceral function that we able to directly control. We can learn to affect other visceral functions such as our heart rate or our blood pressure, but we are not able to directly control them. This voluntary control of breath is important because breathing is the link between our inner and outer

> *We can change our breathing patterns and habitual reactions because we have voluntary control of the breathing mechanism.*

experiences. We take air from the outside world into the body with every inhalation. It is also the link between the physical and emotional reactions we have to those experiences. In other words, what is happening within our bodies and minds is shown by our breathing – even our dreams affect our breath. Conversely, it means that the way we breathe can also change what is happening within our bodies and minds.

We can think of the control of our breathing as existing along a continuum, at one end of the pole it is entirely controlled by the body to the other end, being entirely controlled by the mind. This continuum shows that breathing is the dynamic link between the mind and the body. It spans our physical needs as well as our emotional reactions: it represents our whole experience in the body.

Two Types of Voluntary Breathing – Thoracic and Abdominal

Western medicine recognizes two types of breathing patterns. They correlate with the area of the body where the breathing occurs, and are called thoracic and abdominal breathing. Thoracic refers to the thorax, an area of the chest encased by the ribs. Abdominal refers to the area below the diaphragm, or around the navel. Learning the differences between the two types of breathing is fundamental to improving your health through better breath control.

When we are at rest, abdominal breathing is generally considered the healthiest pattern. It mostly relies upon the contraction and relaxation of the muscle beneath the lungs called the diaphragm. The diaphragm pulls air into the lower part of the lungs. When a body needs more oxygen - such as when exercising, the body may involuntarily supplement abdominal breathing with thoracic breathing, pulling air into the upper part of the lungs.

Thoracic breathing uses the accessory breathing muscles in the upper chest and rib cage rather than the diaphragm. It is shallower and faster than abdominal breathing, and often includes active or forced exhalation. The passive relaxation of the diaphragm is accompanied by active contraction of additional muscles that forces the air out of the lungs, rather than simply allowing the diaphragm to relax, as during abdominal breathing. In other words, in thoracic breathing, we are contracting muscles to exhale, rather than just allowing a contracted muscle to relax.

You can experience these two styles of breathing with the following exercise: [refer figure 1]

Place one hand on your naval and the other hand on your heart. Now take a deep breath. Feel your rib cage elevate and expand - that is thoracic breathing. Now take in a deep breath but concentrate on not moving your rib cage. Instead, slightly push your stomach out into your hand. Try to breathe so that the hand placed over your heart does not move. This is abdominal breathing. Repeat this a few times, exploring the subtleties of the muscle groups working, until you can feel the difference.

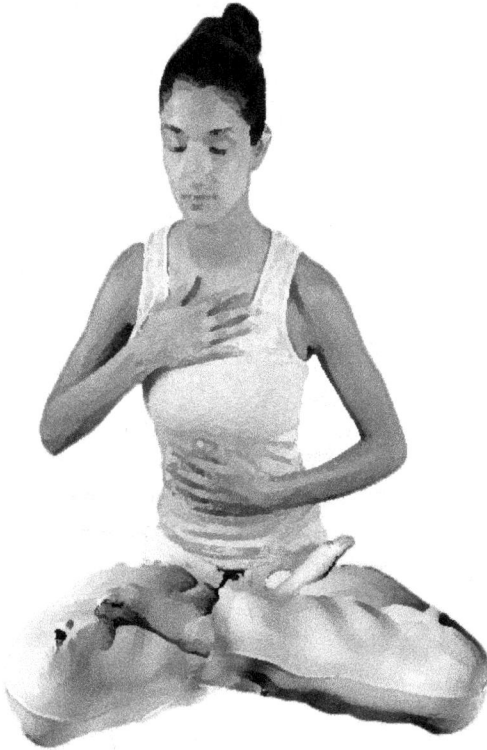

Figure 1
Discovering Abdominal Breathing

The Physical organs of the respiratory system

It is time to examine in more detail how our body works to enable breathing - the actors in this breathtaking drama!

The nose and pharynx

The nose is divided into two nostrils by a nasal septum. The nostrils are lined with mucous membranes that serve to moisten the air and filter out any heavy particles that might become trapped and may be harmful to the internal organs. The nostrils are also lined with a single layer of cells, containing small hair like projections called cilia that act to change the direction of the airflow and heighten its speed. The breath passes through a series of pathways in the nose that act like turbines to increase the speed and direct the flow of the breath toward the deeper lobes of the lungs. They also permit a warming of the air immediately before entering the pharynx on the way to the trachea.

Most *Yogic* breathing exercise require the use of the nose, rather than mouth, because with mouth breathing, the mucous membranes in the throat dry out, increasing the risk of irritation and infection. Become aware of the difference between mouth and nostril breathing. Which is easier and more natural?

The pharynx is a muscular tube that lies behind the nose and mouth, opening into the larynx in front, and the esophagus [the food channel] in the back. The muscles of the pharynx are used chiefly for swallowing.

Larynx

This is composed of pieces of cartilage , and in particular on top is a small piece called epiglottis which closes the passage during swallowing allowing the food to pass into the food canal rather than the trachea or wind-pipe.

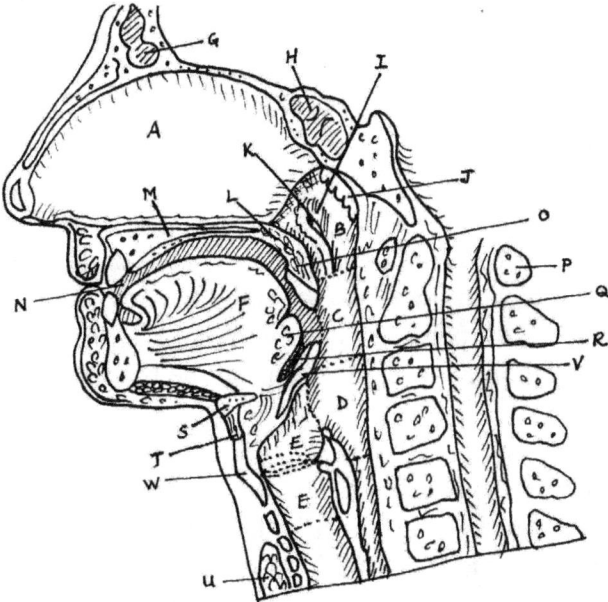

Figure 2
Nasal Cavity and Trachea

A Nasal Septum
B Nasophrynx
C Orophrynx
D Laryngophrynx
E Larynx
F Tongue

G Frontal Sinus
H Sphenoidal sinus
I Tubal tonsil
J Phryngeal tonsil
K Opening of auditory
L Soft palate
M Hard palate

N Oral Cavity
O Uvula
P Spine
Q Lingual tonsil
R Vallecula
S Hyoid Bone
T Thyrohyoid Mrmbtsnr

U Throid Gland
V Epiglottis
W Thyroid
   Cartilage

Vocal Chords

There are two pairs of mucous membrane folds in the larynx. The lower or inferior folds are the true vocal folds or cords. The upper or superior folds are the false vocal cords. Only the true cords create sound, vibrating like violin strings in the air stream. The glottis consists of the true cords and the opening between them. By constricting the glottis, a variable amount of air pass through the voice box.

Trachea

This is a pipe formed by an incomplete ring of cartilages, about 4 inches long, which divides into the right and left bronchi, leading to the lungs. The trachea has to maintain a degree of plasticity under varying thoracic pressures during the breathing process.

Bronchi

The right bronchus divides into three branches and enter into three lobes of the right lung, while the left bronchus divides into two branches to enter the two lobes of the left lung. The most important part of the bronchus is the thin circular layer of smooth muscle which runs all around it. When this muscle contracts, the bronchial passage is restricted, and when it relaxes, the passage is expanded.

The lungs and the alveoli or air sacs

The two lungs fill the chest cavity, separated in the middle by the heart and its blood vessels. They are pear shaped, with smaller upper lobes and larger lower lobes. The upper lobes can extend. The lower lungs are wider than the upper lungs when viewed from the front, and they fill the entire width of the middle rib cage. The bottoms of the lungs are concave, conforming to the shape of the diaphragm's dome.

It is at the single layer of cells in the alveoli that the blood comes into closest contact with the air. Oxygen diffuses from the inhaled air in the air sac into the slowly moving blood circulating around the air sacs.

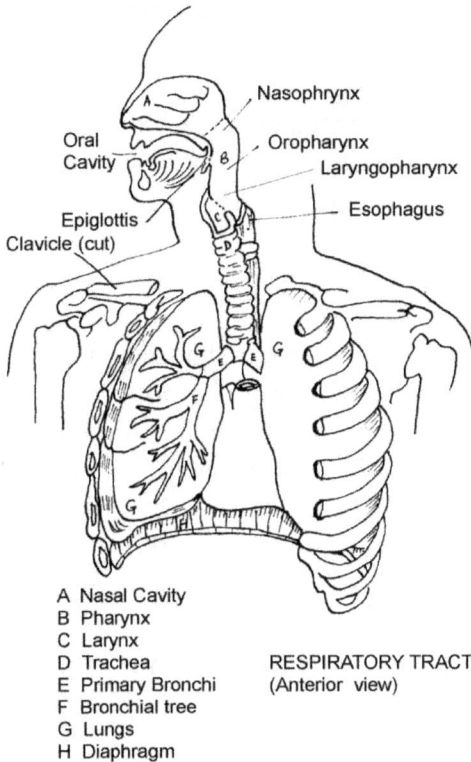

A Nasal Cavity
B Pharynx
C Larynx
D Trachea
E Primary Bronchi
F Bronchial tree
G Lungs
H Diaphragm

RESPIRATORY TRACT
(Anterior view)

Figure 3
. Respiratory Tract: Anterior View

The diaphragm and intercostals muscles

The diaphragm is the domed-shaped sheet of muscle lining the floor of the chest cavity. Contraction of the diaphragm enlarges the chest cavity in the downward direction.

The Intercostal muscles are two oblique strips of muscle in-between the ribs. Contraction of these muscles causes the elevation of the rib-cage and the expansion of the chest outward.

The muscles of the neck attached to the clavicles also play a part in the breathing process. The contraction of these muscles pull up the sternum and clavicle to expand the chest in the upward direction.

Figure 4 shows that the diaphragm divides the heart and lungs from the digestive organs below it. It is the major muscle of respiration. This large flat muscle is shaped somewhat like a full parachute or a dome. The diaphragm's motion is similar to that of a piston, just as the lungs are similar to a combustion chamber. During inhalation, the diaphragm contracts and moves downward, pulling air inward. During shallow breathing, air does not enter the lungs' larger lower regions, while with a full inhalation, air reaches into the lower lungs, where there is more space to receive the full capacity of respiration. During exhalation, the diaphragm relaxes upward and back to its dome shape, allowing for the release of carbon dioxide and other metabolic waste gases.

With *Yogic* breathing, the three sets of muscles, the diaphragm, intercostals and neck muscles, will be strengthened to enable more air to move in and out during a normal respiratory cycle. Thus, the effects of *breath* training will last throughout the day. The quantity of circulating air (called the tidal volume) is increased and the number of breaths per minute is decreased, leading to the development of a more efficient respiratory system.

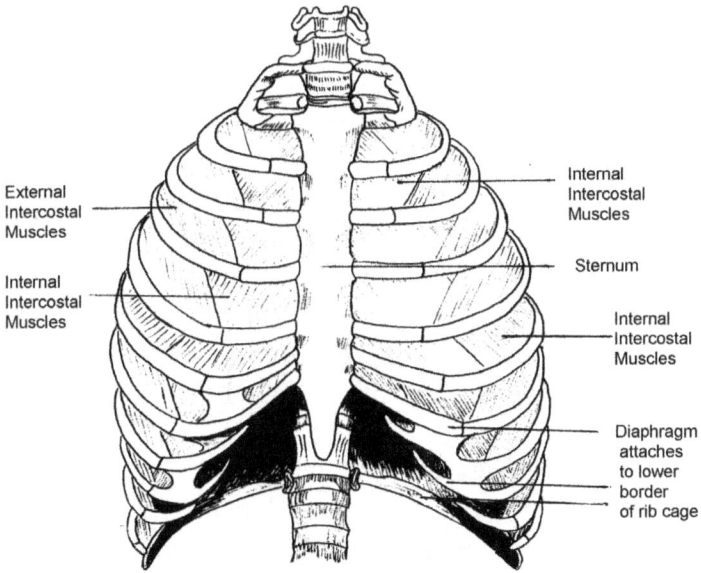

External Intercostal Muscles

Internal Intercostal Muscles

Internal Intercostal Muscles

Sternum

Internal Intercostal Muscles

Diaphragm attaches to lower border of rib cage

Figure 4.
Diaphragm and Intercostal muscles

Learn Abdominal Breathing

We seem to take proper breathing for granted. It is neither taught by parents at home, nor by teachers in schools. In actuality, we all develop bad breathing habits, which can lead to ill-health, but our medical authorities are too focused on prescribing expensive, quick-acting drugs, which work to relieve the symptoms, but do not address the cause of the problems. The best present you can give yourself is learning how to breathe better!

We will start by exploring our breath and breathing patterns. The key to optimizing one's influx of oxygen and life-force is through abdominal breathing. You will be able to look out for the incorrect methods of exhalation and inhalation, while learning the correct method. This abdominal breathing also reduces stress and increases calmness and peace of mind, by lowering the heart rate.

In teaching and advising many students on breathing techniques over the years, there is a consistent reluctance among both men and women to expand their abdomen during inhalation. It seems to be driven by our anxieties over having an extended abdomen. Our popular culture applauds and hungers after a flat, 'washboard' abdomen. You will be glad to know that the proper healthy breathing techniques do not contribute to 'beer-belly'. Rather, the Full *Yogic* Breath, which will be introduced later in the chapter, helps to tone your abdominal muscles.

It is amazing and gratifying to observe the improvements in the quality of life among those who spend just fifteen minutes a day on improving their breath awareness.

Find a comfortable, preferably carpeted floor, and put a sheet on it. Lie down on the floor on your back, relax, and observe the motion of your breath. Let your hands rest at your sides, palms facing up, and with legs separated enough to relax your lower back. Begin by observing your natural breathing pattern. Be mindful of the air as it enters your nostrils.

As you inhale, watch where it expands, and as you exhale, watch where it releases. Be aware of the rate and pace of your breath, and the difference between inhalation and exhalation. Your breathing pattern may vary at different times of the day. Many factors contribute to your breathing pattern, as you will find out, once you relax and become more aware. Some of the major factors which affect breathing, include emotion, physical activity and mental state.

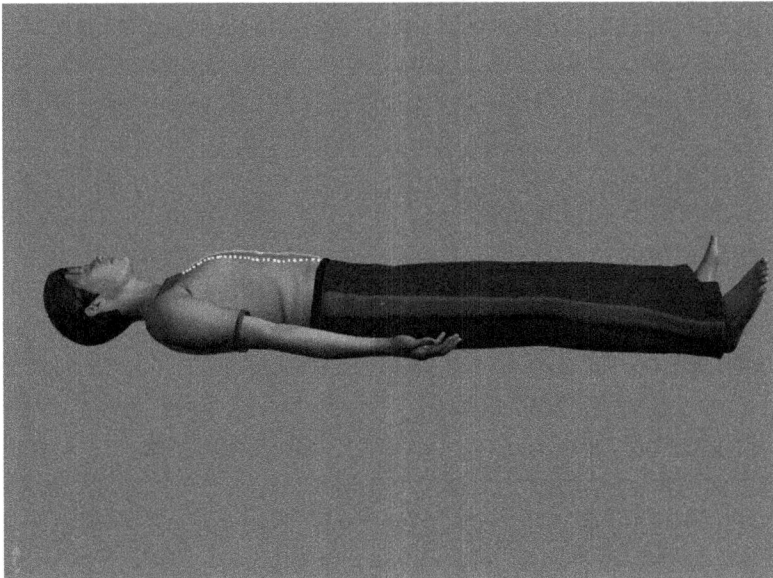

Figure 5:
Abdominal Breathing: Lying down

Feel the interior spaces as your breath enters your head and begins its interior journey down through your trachea into your lungs. Become aware of where you feel the natural motions of your breathing. Does it feel labored or effortless? Do you notice one particular area receiving the breath more than some other regions? You may also be able to distinguish a temperature difference between the inhalation and the exhalation as it moves through your nostrils.

Now focus on your abdominal area, allowing a gentle expansion there as you inhale. Then let it contract and sink inward as you exhale. It is useful to place your hands on your lower abdomen and gently compress your abdominal muscles as you exhale.

When pressure is applied to the middle abdomen during exhalation, a parasympathetic reflex is activated, which will decrease the heart rate and lower blood pressure. The pressure on the abdomen is picked up by a sensor in the aorta which in turn signals the hypothalamus in the mid-brain. The hypothalamus is responsible for regulating heart rate and blood pressure. You will find that abdominal breathing is an effective method to relax.

Continue this abdominal breathing for at least five minutes, to fully feel the calming effect, and benefit from stress relief.

Next, during inhalation, after the expansion of the abdomen, focus on the chest area, and feel the movement of the ribs, outward and upward. Feel the chest expand, with the inhalation, and compress, with the exhalation. Co-ordinate the abdominal breathing with the chest breathing, in a smooth movement, without jerks or strain.

Perform this breathing pattern for at least five minutes, before getting up, off the ground.

After this experience of abdominal breathing lying down, you are ready to observe the same movement in a sitting position. Sit at the edge of a chair, and focus on the abdominal area, expanding it as you inhale, and compressing it as you exhale.

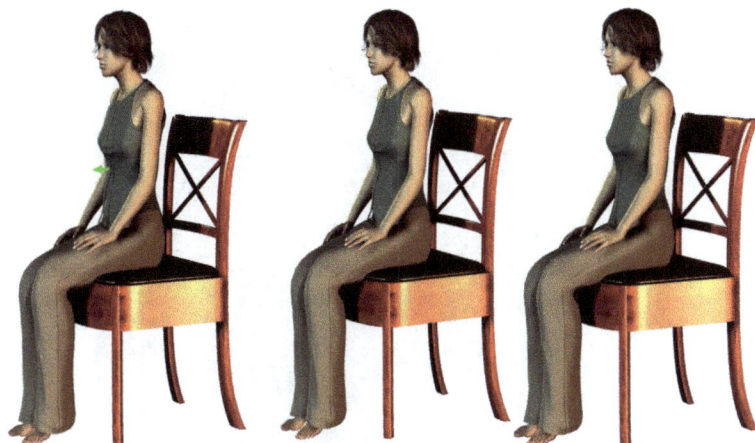

Figure 6:
Abdominal Breathing: sitting position

The next stage in breath awareness is to observe and visualize the movement of the diaphragm that separates the chest from the abdomen, and applying the correct abdominal control.

Inhale: Your diaphragm goes down as air rushes into your lungs. The action of the diaphragm widens your rib cage and also pushes your intestines downward and forward.

Figure 7A shows the incorrect way, because it lets the abdomen move outwards like a balloon. There is no pressure placed on the internal organs, and there may be congestion due to too much blood accumulating in the viscera.

Figure 7B shows the correct abdominal breath. After the diaphragm has reached its lowest position, the abdominal muscles provide a counter pressure. There is no abnormal swelling or deformation of the abdomen. It is held in with a slight pressure.

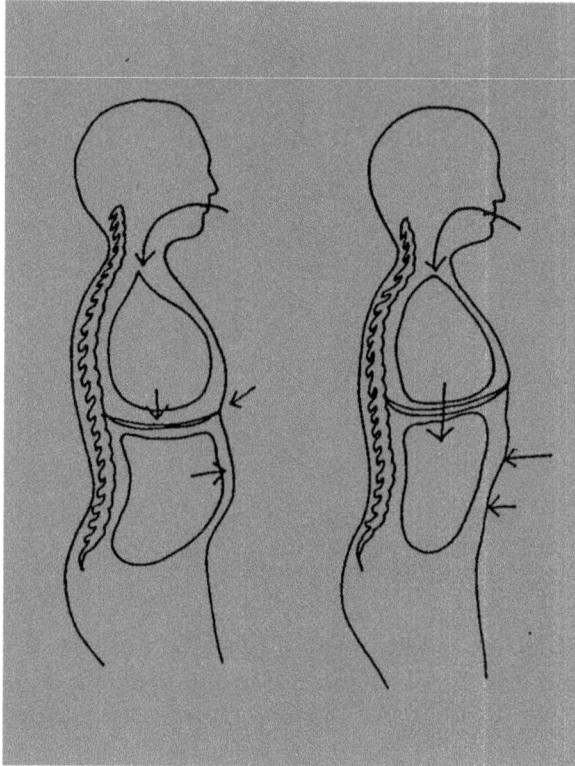

7A   7B
Figure 7:
Incorrect [7A] and Correct [7B] Inhalation

Exhale: Your diaphragm returns to its original position, and air is expelled from your lungs. Your abdomen withdraws and moves up when you breathe out.

Without abdominal control during this phase, the organs are not compressed, since the abdominal muscles are passively following the exhalation. This is an incorrect way to exhale. The correct way is to contract the abdominal muscles at the end of exhalation, consciously pushing the internal organs upwards, expelling the maximum residual air. The diaphragm is pulled up during the exhalation.

Unfortunately, many people do not breathe in the manner that has been described. Instead they swell the belly during exhalation and contract the abdomen during inhalation. This reverse breathing is due to the exaggerated use of the chest, neck, and shoulders. This breathing pattern often causes chronic tension in the neck and shoulders and irregular biological rhythms – menstrual flow, frequent urination, and insomnia. Figure 9 gives another view of the correct control of the diaphragm with the abdominal breathing - it becomes more of an exercise of the diaphragm then of the abdomen.

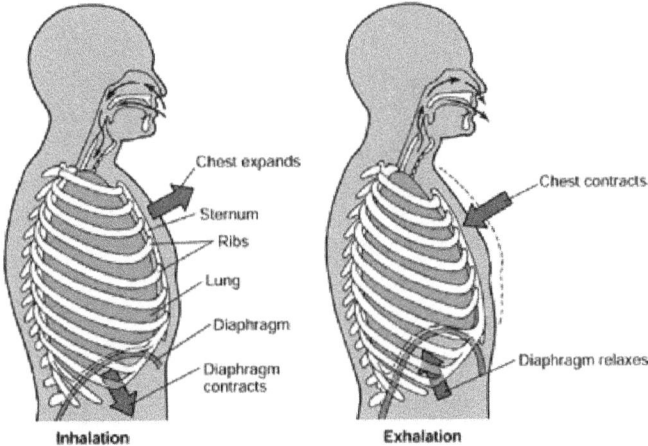

Chest expands
Sternum
Ribs
Lung
Diaphragm
Diaphragm contracts
Inhalation

Chest contracts
Diaphragm relaxes
Exhalation

Figure 8:
Correct Inhale and Exhale

When people regain their natural pattern of abdominal breathing, most of the symptoms of chronic stress fade away. This healing effect of stress relief, is not only due to the decrease in neck and shoulder strain, and the increase in oxygen to the lungs, but also to the increase in *prana* or life-force, which is carried by the breath. Part Two will cover the details about the control and extension of this *prana*.

However, changing deficient breathing patterns require persistent practice, and not only a superficial understanding of the breathing mechanism. Once you've experienced the best way to breathe, putting it into practice will be the goal of the rest of this chapter.

Control of Breathing

In order to understand the mechanism of breathing, it will be useful to understand the chemical control of the process. Although we can breathe without knowing anything about the mechanics, for fuller control and rectification of any bad habits, such knowledge is helpful.

Respiration is regulated and controlled by the nervous system, as well as by the chemical balance in the blood.

The respiratory center is a group of nerve cells in the medulla oblongata, situated in the lower part of the brain stem. This center maintains the basic automatic respiratory reflex. However, it is influenced by the Hypothalamus, which controls the whole autonomic nervous system. Emotional impulses can cause the Hypothalamus to signal to the medulla oblongata to increase the rate and depth of the breath. The frontal cortex of the brain also has a connection to the medullar center for the voluntary control of the breath.

Chemical changes in the blood will signal to the medullar center to change the breathing rate. Too much carbon dioxide and insufficient oxygen will stimulate an increase in the rate and depth of breathing.

As you know from experience, the rate and depth of respiration changes increase with exercise and decrease with rest. The normal rate varies with age, and gender, with a higher rate for younger people and women. It varies from the 10-20 times/minute for an adult to the 40 times per minute of a new-born baby.

For those with good physical and mental health, abdominal and thoracic breathing work together to ensure optimal support for the body - if we need an immediate short-term energy boost, thoracic breathing supports this increase and when we are at rest, abdominal breathing is more efficient since it is slower, deeper, and more calming to the body and mind. Thoracic breathing is inherently less efficient while abdominal breathing has a positive, and cumulative health effects.

Since we need abdominal breathing for the long-term health of the body, its absence will indicate an absence of health or the presence of a medical condition. Results from medical research shows that people who are ill take more thoracic breaths even when at rest than people who are healthy - some medical conditions, such as heart disease, asthma, cancer, and cystic fibrosis, are associated with higher breathing rates with patients breathing in two to three times more air in a minute than healthy people. There are also reports that excessive thoracic breathing is quite common, suggesting that a majority of ambulance runs in major US cities were to provide medical care for persons suffering from symptoms directly related to hyperventilation.

When we breathe in excess of the metabolic demands of the body, we stress the accessory breathing muscles, that is, the muscles in the shoulder girdle as well as the chest wall, while only filling the upper lungs quickly with air. Unfortunately, oxygen exchange is less efficient in the upper lungs. The lower lungs are six

> *Excessive thoracic breathing decreases both oxygen and carbon dioxide in the blood*

to seven times more efficient at exchanging oxygen for carbon dioxide, due to gravity, which pulls the blood supply into the lower lungs, giving more time for oxygen and carbon dioxide to exchange. Therefore upper lung breathing provides the body with less oxygen than breathing with the lower lungs.

You might think that thoracic breathing is beneficial if it reduces the amount of carbon dioxide in the blood, but that would be a mistake. It actually deprives the organs of much needed oxygen because carbon dioxide is necessary for oxygen to be released within the bloodstream, and it is also an important vasodilator; it opens the blood vessels so that blood can flow through. A lack of carbon dioxide causes the smooth muscle in the digestive tract and connective tissue to contract, which restricts blood flow. When the blood vessels constrict, the blood is unable to carry the necessary amount of oxygen to the organs and brain, and the heart also has to work harder to circulate blood throughout the body. When we breathe too shallowly and too rapidly, carbon dioxide is exhaled faster than it is produced, and carbon dioxide levels in the blood decrease. Even though it seems like we are getting more oxygen into our bodies when we breathe rapidly, we are not.

There is also evidence that proper breathing helps the blood and the whole body to maintain a healthy acid/alkai or pH balance, which is necessary for our well-being. Too little carbon dioxide in the blood results in a higher blood pH leading to a medical condition called respiratory alkalosis. If blood pH is out of balance, in this case too alkaline, that imbalance spreads throughout the body compromising its ability to sustain our body's overall health. Respiratory alkalosis can lead to many chronic health conditions that affect the heart and lungs.

Moreover, it is well-known that the proper function of our body cells the cells is dependent on the amount of oxygen they get. It is believed that reduced cell oxygenation is the main cause many chronic diseases and may even encourages the growth of cancerous tumors. As you can imagine, when the cells in the heart-muscles are deprived of oxygen, heart problems can result. Even such diseases as gastrointestinal disorders, diabetes, cystic fibrosis, asthma and bronchitis, have been associated with low amounts of oxygen in the brain or other bodily organs.

On the flip side, deep abdominal breathing promotes full exchange of oxygen for carbon dioxide and so does not cause the health problems associated with shallow thoracic breathing. In fact, it can slow the heartbeat and lower or stabilize blood pressure which are all good signs for overall health and well-ness.

The Physical health benefits of Breath Training and Therapy

When you watch an infant sleeping, it is easy to determine that it is breathing primarily by using the diaphragm because you can see the abdomen rise and fall, with each breath. It would stand to reason that teaching chronically ill adults to practice diaphragmatic breathing, rather than habitual chest pattern breathing, could restore their health, given what we have discussed so far about the oxygenation benefits of the Complete Breath.

Indeed, researches in China, India and Russia have shown that over 90% of the patients with peptic ulcers can be successfully treated with breathing exercises. Russian research [Kreme Sanatorium] has also have shown successful treatment of tuberculosis patients, while Indian research supports the treatment of patients with hypertension.

Much more research, especially in the United States would be needed to uncover all the potential health benefits of Breath Training and Therapy.

However, we do not need to wait for the results from modern researchers to confirm the insights of thousands of years of yogic science, or what can be confirmed by your own efforts for a few weeks!

A Summary of the types of Breathing

The ancient masters of breath have classified four different methods of breathing:

- Abdominal or diaphragmatic or low breathing
- Intercostal or middle breathing
- Clavicular or upper breathing
- Complete *Yogic* breathing

Abdominal Breathing consists of the movement of the diaphragm and of the outer wall of the abdomen. As you inhale the diaphragm muscle is flattened from a dome shape to a disc shape, as it moves downwards. This compresses the abdominal organs and eventually pushes the front wall, the navel and the abdomen outwards. This movement acts as a massage to the upper abdominal organs, such as liver, stomach, transverse large intestine, and pancreas. With practice, it will also massage the mid-abdominal organs,particularly, the ascending and descending large intestine and the centrally located small intestines. The abdominal muscles must relax for this to occur, causing a slight swelling of the belly. A counter pressure from the abdomen is applied, once the diaphragm has reached its maximum position.

As you exhale, the abdominal muscles contract more and the diaphragm moves upwards, reducing the volume in the chest cavity, and relaxing back into a dome shape, mildly compressing the lungs and heart. The contractions during abdominal breathing tone the centrally located rectus abdominis muscle, strengthening it to move more air in and out, and increasing the quantity of air circulating within the body (called the tidal volume) and reducing the number of breaths per minute. Abdominal breathing is physiologically the most efficient because it draws in the greatest amount of air for the least amount of muscular effort.

In Intercostal Breathing, the movement of the ribs becomes the focus. The rib movements are caused by two sets of muscles between the ribs: the internal and external intercostals. These muscles depress and narrow the rib cage during exhalation. During inhalation, the intercostals reverse the process to expand the rib cage's diameter, increasing the internal cavity space to allow the lungs to expand, resulting in air being drawn down into them from the front side..

In Clavicular Breathing, inhalation and deflation of the lungs is achieved by raising the upper ribs, shoulders and collarbones (clavicles). Very little air is inhaled and exhaled, since this movement cannot change the volume of the chest cavity very much, requiring maximum effort to obtain minimum benefit.

This upper breathing is common in our society, owing to the modern lifestyles we have adopted in the cities where we are subjected to stressful conditions – noise, pollution, badly ventilated rooms and offices, as well as second-hand smoke. The competitive work arena contributes further to the state of anxiety, immobilizing the diaphragm in an attempt to deal with the deep-seated fears of aggression and other deep emotional feelings, causing harmful shallow breathing.

Complete natural or *Yogic* Breathing combines all the above three methods of breathing into one complete harmonious movement. The entire respiratory system is brought into full use, exercising all the respiratory muscles including the internal and external intercostals and abdominal muscles, as well as the rib cage, the lungs and their air sacs, and the diaphragm. Our goal should be to develop this type of complete breathing which can give the maximum benefit for the body.

Breathing Exercise No. 1: The Complete Breath

Sit in a comfortable posture, either cross-legged on the floor or at the edge of a chair, with the spine straight, but without unnecessary tension. All breathing should be performed through the nostrils and not through the mouth, in a warm and well-ventilated room.

This is divided into four parts. In the first three parts, we exercise the separate muscles for the breath, while in the fourth part, we combine all three together in a smooth breathing movement.

Part 1
Abdominal and diaphragmatic breathing

Place the palms of your hands lightly on your abdomen. This is to make you aware of the movement in your abdomen as the air is breathed in and out of the lowest lobes of your lungs. Breathe out slowly and completely, becoming aware of the movement of your diaphragm that is responsible for your abdominal breathing. As you exhale, feel your abdomen contract and your navel moving back towards the spine. At the end of exhalation the diaphragm will be totally relaxed and will be doming or parachuting upwards into the chest cavity.

Now, inhale, keeping your chest and shoulders still. Expand the abdomen and feel the navel moving outwards and upwards. The breathing should be deep and slow. At the end of the inhalation your diaphragm will be bowing in the direction of the abdomen and your navel will be as high as it can move.

Exhale again, slowly and completely, contracting the abdomen. Then without any holding of breath, inhale and then repeat the whole process twice more, for a total of three abdominal breaths.

Now move your hands around to your back, so that your palms are resting on your lower back, with the fingers pointing towards the spine. Perform three more abdominal breaths, concentrating your mind on the movement of the lungs, as sensed by your lightly resting hands.

Part 2
Intercostal and lower rib breathing

We will now exercise the intercostals muscles. Throughout this practice, keep the abdomen still by slightly contracting the abdominal muscles.

Place your hand on either side of the middle rib cage, so that the fingers of each palm are pointing towards each other. This will help you feel the expansion and contraction of the ribs. Remember that the intercostals are the muscles between the ribs.

Inhale slowly by expanding the rib cage outwards and upwards. You will find it impossible to breathe deeply because of the limitation on the maximum expansion of the chest.

Slowly exhale by contracting the chest downwards and inwards. Keep the abdomen slightly contracted, but without strain
.

Breathe in slowly, repeating the whole process two more times
.

Now, place your hands behind the mid-area of your back, opposite to where you had your hands placed on your front. Concentrate and breathe into the middle back area using the rib muscles for another three rounds.

Part 3
Clavicular or upper breathing

In this exercise, try your best not to move the abdomen or the intercostals, keeping them slightly contracted, but immobile.

Place both palms on your upper chest, so that you can determine whether your chest is moving or not, while trying not to contract the muscles of your abdomen. Inhale by drawing your collarbones and shoulders upwards towards your chin, similar to a shrugging movement. If you have difficulty with this movement, try to inhale and exhale with a sniffing action, which automatically induces upper breathing.

Exhale by letting your shoulders and collarbones move downwards away from your chin.

Do this clavicular breathing two more times.

Now, raise your arms over your shoulders, and breathe deeply and slowly into the upper lobes of the lungs, feeling the movement and breath under the armpits.

Perform this three times with concentration and awareness, but without strain.

Part 4
The Complete Breath

This is a combination of the three previous exercises, taking the maximum volume of air into the lungs and expelling the maximum amount of carbon dioxide.

Breathe out deeply, contracting the abdomen to squeeze all the air from the lungs. It is important in this exercise to maintain control in a smooth manner without jerkiness. Each part should transition into the next imperceptibly.

Now, inhale slowly, keeping the lowest part of the abdomen slightly contracted, while expanding the part above the navel. The slight contraction of the lowest abdomen is to help you get over the fear of getting a pot-belly due to the abdominal organs moving down.

At the end of the upper abdomen expansion, start to expand your chest and rib cage outwards and upwards. Continue drawing the breath upwards into the higher lobes of your lungs by raising your collarbones and shoulders towards your chin. Your lungs should now be completely filled with air.

Then, without holding your breath or interrupting the continuous nature of the breathing pattern, begin to exhale, first relaxing your collarbones and shoulders. Then allow your chest to move first downwards and then inwards. Finally, contract the abdomen. Do not strain but try to empty your lungs as much as possible, squeezing all the air out by drawing the abdominal wall closer to the spine.

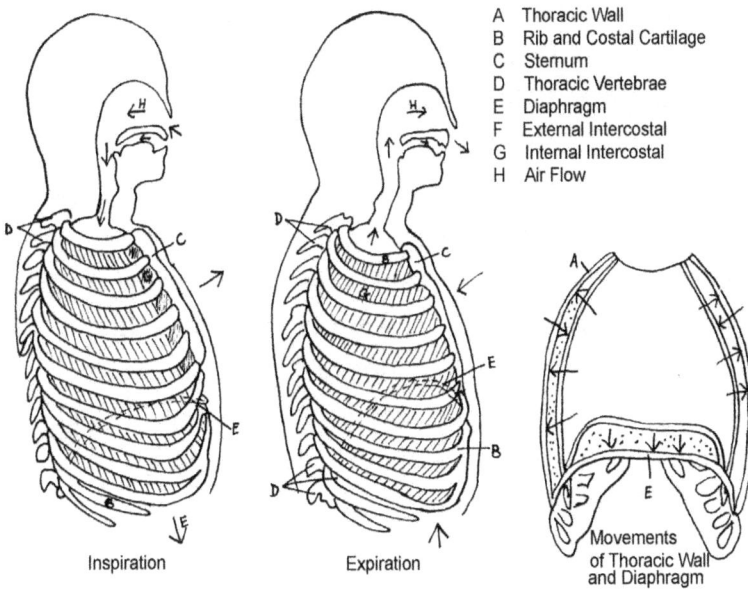

A   Thoracic Wall
B   Rib and Costal Cartilage
C   Sternum
D   Thoracic Vertebrae
E   Diaphragm
F   External Intercostal
G   Internal Intercostal
H   Air Flow

Inspiration   Expiration   Movements of Thoracic Wall and Diaphragm

Figure 9: Complete Yogic Breath Movement

This completes one round of *The Complete Breath* cycle. Continue for another six rounds. If you need to rest between the rounds, you may take a few "normal" breaths, before continuing.

Practice this breathing exercise for ten minutes, twice a day for the next two weeks, and observe the changes in your energy level. Make this breathing pattern your daily routine, if you observe increase in your energy level and reduction in stress. Your quality of life will be markedly improved when you adopt The Complete Breath as your daily wake-up recipe, rather than relying on that cup of coffee!

The Complete Breath should be one continuous movement, each phase of breathing merging into the next, without there being any physical jerks, strain or even obvious transition point. The body should remain relaxed throughout the practice.

After some practice you will find that this Complete Breath will become second nature to you. Begin to develop the habit of consciously breathing whenever you can throughout the day. If you feel tired, depressed, angry or anxious, then center yourself, sit down, and practice this technique. Breathe deeply and slowly with your concentration on the breath. Feel that you are inhaling not just air, but courage, strength, and peace. As you exhale, breathe away any negative qualities that your mind may be holding on to. Then your mind will become calm and revitalized

Besides the emotional and mental benefits, the Complete Breath develops good healthy lung tissues that resist germs, making you much less susceptible to disease. The blood receives plenty of oxygen and every organ of the body is nourished by it. Digestion and assimilation are improved, and bodily energy and vigor are increased.

Stress: The Destroyer of happiness and good health

What causes stress and why is it bad for our well-being?

Many different factors contribute to our experience of stress. However, fundamentally it is a hormonal and instinctual survival response from our evolutionary origins. It is our response to danger. The release of stress hormones enables us to perform at peak speed and strength. Think about the mother who lifts a car to save her trapped child! The feeling of stress heightens our senses and blood rushes to the major muscles of our arms and legs for immediate physical actions.

On the positive side, stress hormones give us a boost of strength and agility but on the negative side, it throws the body and mind out of balance. Under ordinary circumstances, we physically exert ourselves in order to face a short-term the danger and when the immediate danger is no longer present, the chemicals disperse and the physical and mental systems return to balance.

The deadly problem is that in our modern world, we are seldom faced with the mortal physical dangers of our ancestors and we now perceive most of our harm coming from hidden dangers such as the loss of wealth, health, job security, relationships and such. It is now our mind that is responsible for our stress reactions rather than any physical stimulus. This is dangerous because the mind can continuously trigger our stress response in the absence of any immediate danger and will not let the system return to balance. We are continually stressed out of balance due to our perception of ourselves in this world.

The kind of situations that causes stress these days are countless, from getting cut off in traffic to worrying about the next car-payment to trying to make a good impression of a first date. These stress situations cause problems that don't require a strong physical response but the chemicals released into the blood require a physical activity in order to disperse. If we do not physically exert ourselves to resolve a stressful situation, it takes longer to restore the balance between the sympathetic and parasympathetic nervous systems. What is worse for our well-being is when a stress inducing stimulus is mentally replayed as part of a cyclical thought pattern and then the same stress is perceived over and over again, and the body does not get adequate time to relax, rebalance, and reset itself.

What happens when our body falls out of balance due to stress hormones? Our heart rate increases and we tend to hold our breath. As a result, we are unable to breathe deeply, and we engage in short, shallow thoracic breathing. Thus, the same responses that save us from immediate danger can also suppress the immune system, restrict blood flow, and drain us of physical, mental, and emotional energy.

Factors that contribute to the increase of stress in everyday life:

1. Fast paced life-style in the modern world with technological advances such as rapid transport can cause physical stress.

Danger of stress - increased likelihood of physical illness, anxiety, or depression

Our bodies have not yet adjusted to the new technological age.

2. Emails! Messaging! Mental and emotional stress. It is only two decades since the widespread adoption of the internet but it has already caused a tremendous revolution in life-style habits. Who still remembers how to write a letter? Twitter has condensed all communications to 140 characters. It is not bad per se, but these are all changes that contributes to our stressing out more and more.

3. Vicarious entertainment options such as horror movies and thrill rides

4. In developing countries, people are focused on material survival – food and a roof over their heads. In developed countries, there is less concern for survival and more on satisfying desires and our minds can get consumed by the stress of achieving our desires or losing what our prized possessions.

5. Most of us have to makes many choices in our lives, some important and some trivial. Every day, we are beset with a range of decisions to be made – what clothes to wear? Which restaurant to go for dinner? Which movie to watch? What to get for a loved one's birthday? When to ask for a raise from your boss? When and where to take a vacation? Buy a new car? A new house? A new boy-friend? I'm sure you can fill in more.

> *The Complete Breath in exercise 1 and the new technique called The Calming Breath helps to restore the hormonal balance quickly so as to reduce the over-reactions to stress*

Do you know that all these choices contribute to your stress level? Uncertainty gives rise to stress and worry. Some research indicates that when we suffer from stress and anxiety, the chemical effect on the brain makes it difficult to think clearly and process information related to making choices. The inability to choose is exacerbated by the sheer number of choices available to us which compounds the stress level. Try finding the best brand of cereal in a supermarket and you will soon find yourself mentally exhausted!

7. Increased levels of pollution in contribute to increasing stresses on the body system to flush toxins out. There are also indications that increasing chemical ingredients in our food can also contribute

to lowering the ability of the body to deal with stress.

7. Lack of physical movement: it is not necessary that we should all run the a marathon or even join a gym to work-out. The problem is the avoidance of even the simple exercise of walking instead of driving for a mile or two to the post office or convenience store. A stagnant body accumulates the stress chemicals that need to be flushed out. For good health, some level of exercise is required.

8. Physical rigidity: this is where simple stretches such as yoga asanas can help to improve your well-being. This stiffness and inflexibility of the body is a symptom of stress induced blockages in the nervous system, the muscles and even the subtle energy channels that we will examine more in Part 3 of the book. Maintaining a flexible body is key to reducing the effects of stress by removing these blockages and potential health hazards.

Breathing Exercise 2: The Calming Breath

This is an excellent breathing technique for reducing stress and producing a calm mind. It helps to put the body and mind into a state of ease called 'sukha'. It is simple to learn but should not be dismissed, in favor of more complex breathing techniques. This is a case where simplicity increases effectiveness.

Sit comfortably, keeping a smiling face, and relaxed body. You can use any posture where you can keep your back straight and head aligned without undue tension. Keep eyes closed. Relax your jaw and facial muscles.

Take a deep breath through your nostrils and then hold your breath for about ten seconds. During the hold of breath, tense your whole body as hard as you can. Then turn your head to the left and forcefully exhale out through your mouth. Release all tension. Repeat this cycle two more times.

Once more, relax and put a smile on your face.
Inhale slowly, but without strain from both nostrils, and then exhale slowly through both nostrils. Keep attention on the breath coming in and out of the nostrils at your regular rate of breathing for a few minutes.

Then, follow the breath as you inhale into your body. Be aware of the sensations of the body and find the spot where you start to exhale, following the exhale breath back to the nostrils. Do this for a few minutes to fully immerse yourself in your breath.

Now, feel your body being energized by the breath. Let go of fully of the urge to control the breath. Just let it happen in your awareness. Mentally count the duration of the inhalation and exhalation. Don't try to control the length of either one. After a couple of breaths, try to make the exhalation to be of the same number of counts as the inhalation.

It takes practice to count the duration of your breath, but after a little while, it will be second nature. The key at the beginning is to count consistently, and not vary the speed of the count. Continue for a few minutes.

It is generally recommended that you begin with a count of six, moving to twelve, after several weeks of practice.

Let your awarenss of breath go deeper - after the inhalation or the exhalation, if there is natural pause, don't force the breath, and wait for the continuation. Your respiratory system will take care of it. Continue for a few more minutes before wrapping it up by doing a couple of rounds of Complete Breath

Take the time to learn and practice this Calming Breath. After you are able to perform to a count of twelve, integrate it with exercise 1, The Complete Breath.

Part 2

Our Well-Being
&
The Life-force Energy

What is Life-Force Energy?

There are two sources of energy for the body: indirectly from food and directly from life force. It can take hours to convert food into energy, but the your Will can immediately generate the necessary energy from the Universal Energy reservoir. In order for you to tap into the reservoir you need to understand the nature of the body life force. We will be exploring in much greater depth this life -force in Part 3. For now, we only need to understand how it affects our body, mind and emotions in a general way.

The ancient sages in their quest for knowledge went into deep meditative states. During these states, they discovered that all living beings are surrounded by an energy field which dissipated at death. They called this prana or life-force field.

The sages discovered that the life-force energy fluctuated with the living conditons and health, both physical and emotional, of the person. They found that the breath was intimately connected with the life-force and the quality of the breath greatly affected the energy field.

There is no scientify proof for the existence of the life-force called prana. However, neither has it been disproved by science.

Its presence is validated by personal experience.

The breath is not only a source of support for the physical body; it is also a support for mental, emotional, and spiritual well-being. The mental, emotional, and spiritual aspects of the breath are easily understood in the yogic tradition where the air element is central to all of life - including all of our physical, mental, and spiritual experiences. This air element should not be confused with the normal use of the words air or element. It is meant to denote an universal building block responsible fo material movement. Therefore it would be better to use the technical term vayu.

In the Yogic teachings, vayu and the breath are tied together through the word prana, which is embedded with several layers of meaning. Prana describes not only the breath, the movement of air and the basic atmosphere around us, but it has the additional meaning of "prana energy." From the point of view of Yoga and the practice of meditation, the physical body is permeated by five types of prana energy, which support the body's most basic functions, such as circulation, digestion, and excretion. Therefore, accordingly, the breath is part of an intricate system of prana energy that regulates and supports the body's health. For this reason, we often use the words breath and prana energy interchangeably. However, while the breath is one form of prana energy, referring to prana energy speaks to our entire bodily system, and all of its physical, mental, and emotional components. Yoga tells us that when all the prana energy is in balance, all of the body's basic systems work efficiently and we feel healthy.

So far, we have been speaking of the bodily prana which is responsible for the well-being of the gross and subtle bodies of a being such as a human. However, we also a spiritual prana which permeates a spiritual field around us. This spiritual prana which we shall not be investigation further is providing the engine to power all human beings to the next level of evolution.

We will be concerned in this program only with the physical prana which is affecting our body, mind and emotions. There is prana in our bodies, and there is prana outside our bodies. We are swimming in a sea of prana, which can be absorbed through our breath and through our skin. It is in the food we eat and the sunshine that bathes our skin. There are energy centers in our subtle body which absorbs and stores this prana.

We will be learning two new exercises in the section in order to increase our absorption of prana. This will result in a marked increase in your energy level and awareness. However, in order to sustain and maintain this higher state of well-being, it is necessary for you to drop or avoid situations and habits which can decrease your energy level and put you back into a lower state, in which you mightbe more susceptible to disease. In addition to avoiding life-draining situations, one should cultivate life force enhancing habits and situations.

What are the life force draining habits and situations which should be avoided? What to cultivate?

1. Avoid places which have a lot of negative energy. Our system can get depleted trying to resist and fight off the negativity. Bars, brothels and casinos are examples of places where lust, greed, anger and fear permeate palpably. There are very few places in our modern society where you can find positive energy – try going to different churches, and find one where you feel good after spending some time there.

2. The pollution in our cities deprive us of life-giving prana. Try to spend time in the fresh air of parks and mountains. The amount of prana is directly proportional to the oxygen in the air.

3. Avoid the company of people who have bad habits because they have low energy levels, and will drain you of your higher energy, much like a "vampire". All of us have had the experience of being drained after spending time with someone. This does not mean that we do not bring comfort to those in need, which is a conscious effort to help others. Cultivate the companionship of those who have abundance of positive energy, and who can help you in your path to self-healing.

4. Avoid idle chatter and loose talk. The spoken word is full of energy. There are great masters of yoga who recognizing this had achieved self-realization, in part, by keeping silence for extended periods of time, to build

up their energy level. We do not need to go that far, but some level of control will be beneficial. Sometimes, we feel so excited that we are drawn to share with someone, and feel drained afterwards. It is always best to cultivate a middle path of non-excess.

5.   Avoid over indulgence in sensual pleasures. Eating too much is bad for your health, just as drinking too much, or having too much indiscriminate sex. All these sensual activities will drain you of your Prana. Cultivate a moderate appetite in all things.

All of us have different needs. Each of you must bear the responsibility to implement the kind of healthy life force enhancing plan that appeals to you..

Let us also consider the effect of breath and prana on our emotional well-being. We may think of the breath as something that is simply related to the exchange of oxygen and carbon dioxide and that keeps us alive. However, prana energy not only supports our ordinary bodily systems but it also quite literally drives our emotions. Thus, it is more than simply the experience of inhalation and exhalation. Prana energy is also the physical rush of energy that accompanies all of our feelings and sensations. If we examine the body and mind carefully, we notice a connection between the breath and how we feel. When the breath is calm and relaxed, we notice that the body's energy is also calm, especially in the areas of the abdomen, lungs, and chest. As a result, the mind becomes clear and we feel relaxed and even-tempered. We feel that we can take things as they come and that we are capable of dealing with whatever life brings us.

When we are emotionally upset, we may notice that we breathe harder and faster, or that we are unable to inhale deeply and exhale fully. We notice a sense of pain, heaviness, or dullness in the abdomen and chest area, or even throughout the whole body, and that the mind is agitated by thoughts or overpowered by emotion. This overpowering energy manifests in all sorts of neurotic ways, such as depression, obsession, fear of intimacy, fear of trust, or feelings of grandiosity or inadequacy. In addition, Western medicine connects our psychological state with respiratory alkalosis. Respiratory alkalosis is associated with a lower pain threshold, with feelings of discomfort and agitation, and with imbalances such as anxiety and fatigue—all the result of less efficient oxygen delivery to the tissues and organs, including the brain. Some research states that dysfunctional breathing is as high as 5 to 11 percent in the general population, 30 percent in asthmatics, and up to 83 percent in those who suffer from anxiety.

When putting things in the context of prana energy, all of these emotions are simply an expression of imbalanced prana energy. However, even though all of these states of mind are a sign of unbalanced prana energy, they feel very different. And though the experiences of neurotic mind, energy, and emotions can appear and feel very different from one to the other, in every single case the mind can be thoroughly pacified and calmed through working with the breath.

> *Research has associated breathing patterns with specific emotional states - and it has also shown that we can influence our emotions by the way we breathe.*

Of course, change will not happen immediately. But generally speaking, over a long period of time, working with the breath is effective at cutting through all types of neurotic tendencies, because it brings the prana energy into balance. As the prana energy is brought into balance and becomes more stable, neurotic tendencies lessen and even begin to disappear.

Breathing Exercise Three: The Energy Balance

A tonic to awaken and distribute the life-foce healing energy throughout the body, for releasing physical, emotional and mental blockages. It establishes equanimity and connectedness to the universal source of all energy. This technique can be practiced at any time and is especially effective at sunrise when facing the sun.

- Sit in any comfortable position where you can feel relaxed and balanced. We will be learning more about seating postures in Part 3 but at this time, you can sit on the edge of a chair or cross-legged on the floor. Place the right palm on top of the left palm. Close the eyes and relax the whole body, yet maintaining a straight back.

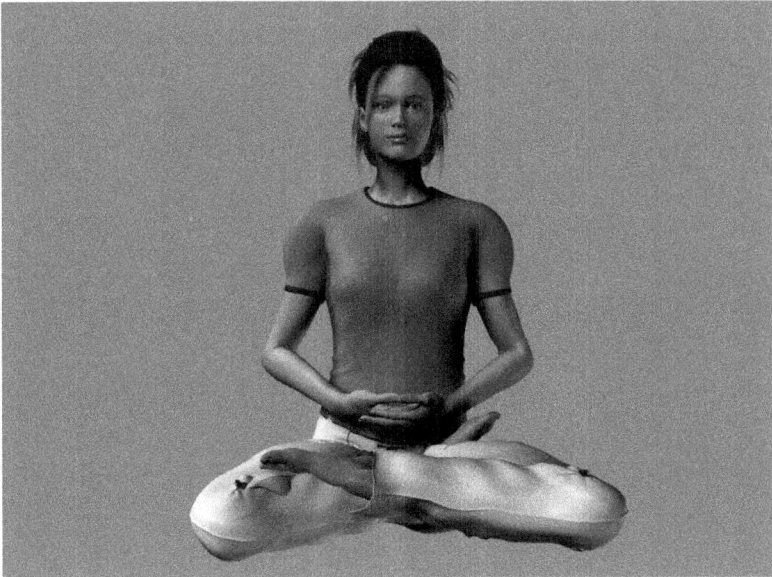

Figure 10: Position 1

- Utilizing the abdominal breathing, inhale and exhale deeply, expelling the maximum amount of air from the lungs, by contracting the abdominal muscles. While the breath is held out for a moment, contract the perineum and the anal sphincter. The perineum is the space between the sexual organs and the anus. It has its own muscle group and can be contracted towards the tailbone. Contracting the perineum and the anal sphincter will be require a little bit of practice. It is the same as contracting any muscular group of the body such as the when you make a fist. The contraction is held lightly and not with great tension.

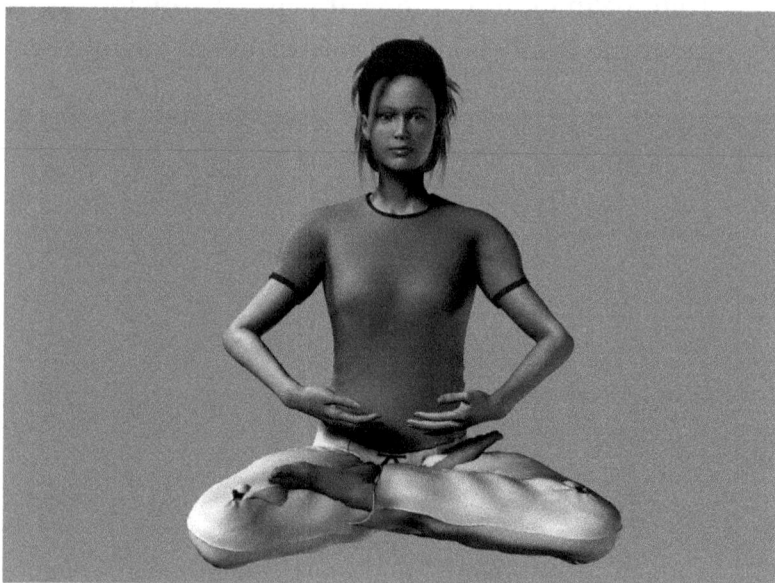

Figure 11: Position 2

- While maintaining this contraction, begin inhaling

slowly, expanding the abdomen fully to draw in the maximum air into the lungs. Push down the diaphragm. At the same time, raise the hands to the level of the navel center. The hands are not touching, with fingers pointing towards each other and the palms facing inwards. There should be no tension in the arms. During the inhalation, feel and visualize the *prana* or life-force being drawn from the *base of the spine* to the *back of the naval* along the spinal column.

- Continue with thoracic breathing, expanding the chest and simultaneously raising the hands to the heart center. Feel the prana rising from the back of the navel to the back of the chest along the spine.

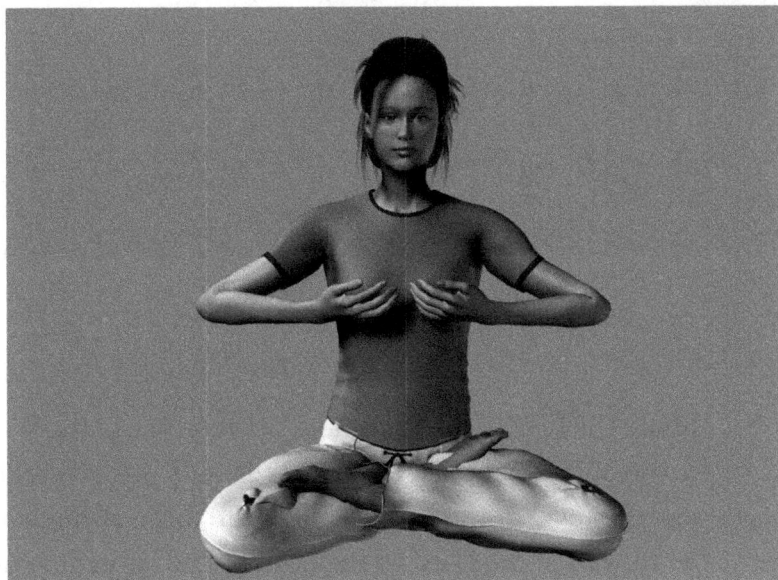

Figure 11: Position 3

- Complete the inhalation with clavicular breathing, raising the shoulders slightly and drawing some more air into the lungs. Feel the life-force energy being drawn from the heart center to the throat center, as you raise your hands to the front of the throat.

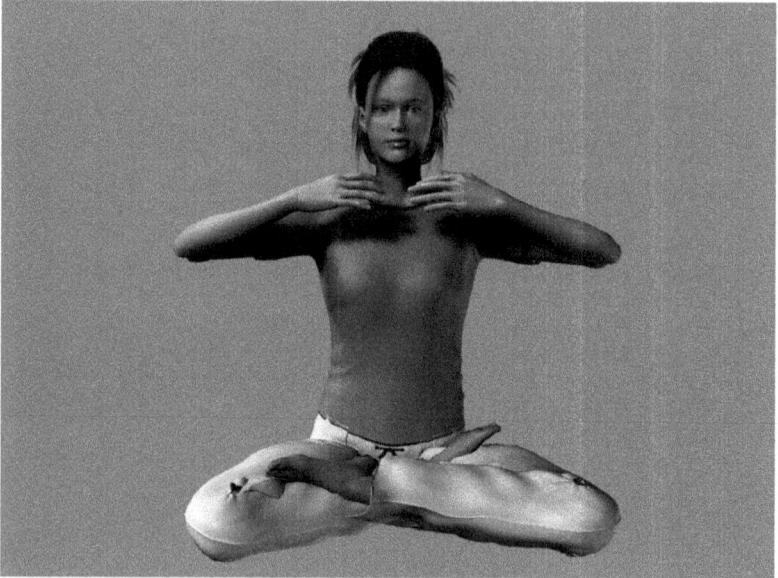

Figure 12: Position 4

- Retain the breath for a moment, as you spread the arms to the sides, palm facing upwards and out-stretched near the level of the ears. Feel the life force rising from the throat up the head to the crown, and spreading out from the top of the head and emanating all around you. At this time you can release the slight contraction lower msucles of the perineum and anus.

[51]

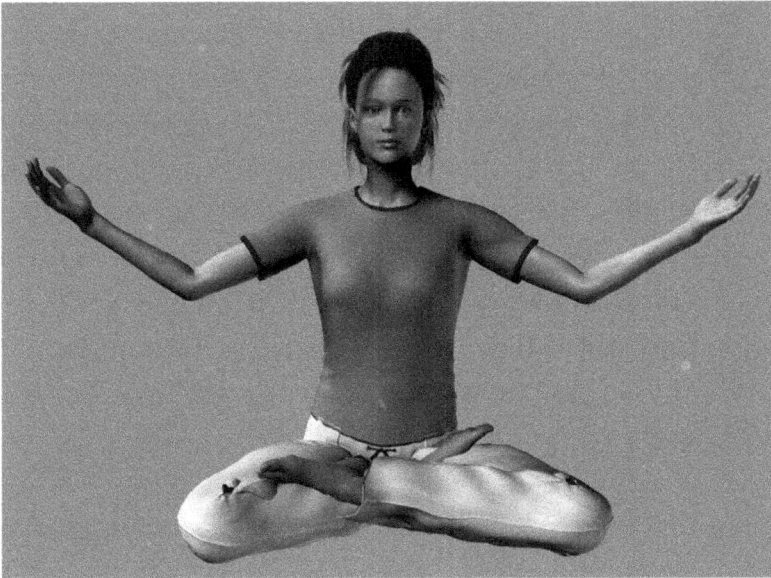

Figure 13: Position 5

- Begin exhalation, by lowering the shoulders and returning the hands to its position in front of the throat, feeling the prana descending to the back of the neck. Contract the chest muscles, and lowering the hands to the heart center, as the prana descends to the back of the heart.. Complete the exhalation by contracting the abdomen, lowering the hands to the navel, as the prana descends to the navel area. At the end of the exhalation, the hands are resting on top of the thighs, as at the beginning of the cycle.

- Repeat twice more and then completely relax.

- There is a supplementary technique for energization that I find extremely powerful to use during the relaxation phase after this energization with breath. It utilizes the deep knowledge that the sages had of our energy field. They found that the fingers of our hands, especially the tips are intimately connected to the activity of our energy system. By touching them together in various ways, they discovered they could affect our energy field. They called these different hand gestures mudras and you can find many statues and paintings from India and China displaying various mudras.

- This Prana Mudra helps to increase the strength of our energy field and boosts the health and vitality of the body. On both hands, bend the little finger and the ring fing to touch their tips together with the tip of the thumb. The index and middle fingers are straightened out. You can hold this mudra for five to ten minutes. You can also use this mudra at other times to remove fatigue.

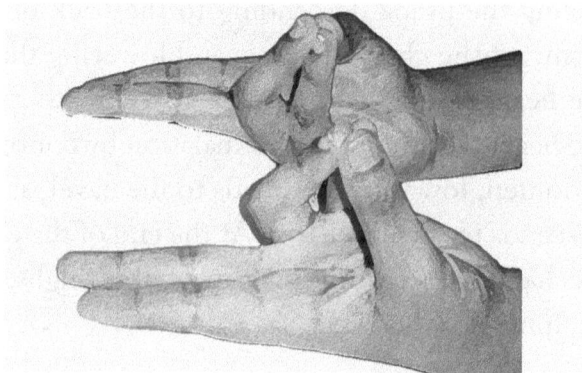

Figure 14: Prana Mudra

Breathing Exercise 4: Dynamic Energy Booster

This is a set of exercises which are very beneficial for energizing the body, as well as opening up the lungs. These are done in the early morning, before the other breathing exercises.

These simple exercises are based on the fact that tensing a muscle, restricts energy flow to it, while relaxing the same muscle, enables energy to flow unimpeded to it. An additional advantage for beginners, is that instead of tensing and relaxing individual muscles, the tension is initiated by pressing a pair of muscles together, isometrically.

The yogis of the Himalayas have pioneered the use of such "isometric" techniques, millennia before the West discovered them. They are generally easier to learn and perform than the traditional yogic postures. This set also stretches and loosens up the spine, for easing the upward flow of energy. They also have the benefit of balancing the body-mind connection.

The key to performing these exercises, is to bring your awareness, into every movement, and to seamlessly integrate your breath with the movements, according to the instructions.

Energization Exercise #1

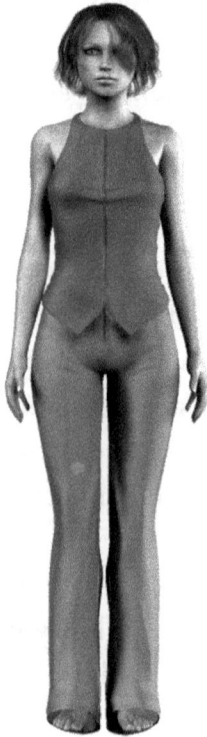

Stand straight with hands by your side. Eyes are softly focused ahead. Become aware of the body. Become aware of the air passing through your nostrils. Feel your feet sink into the floor.

Become aware of different parts of your body. Feel the right hand, the right elbow, the right shoulder, right arm-pit, the right hip, the right knee, the right ankle and the right foot. Repeat with the left side.

Become aware of the face, head and throat. Smile into your eyes.

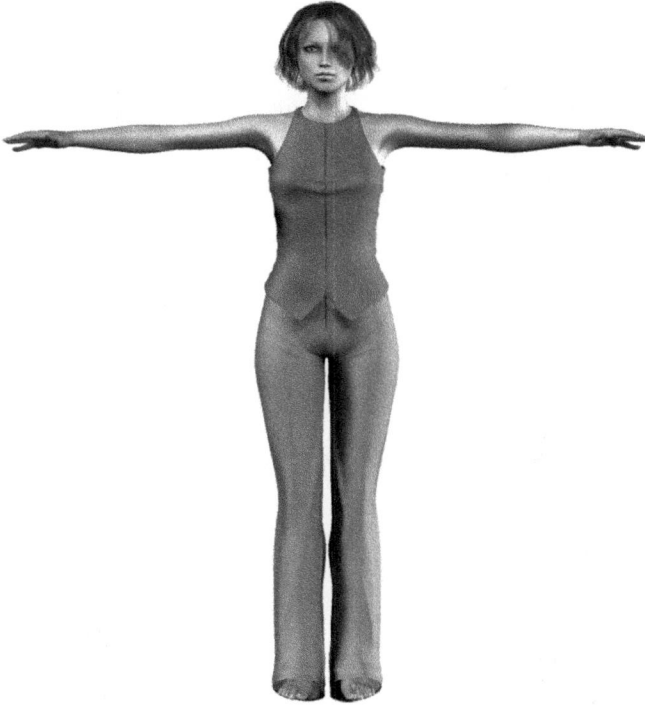

As you inhale slowly through the nostrils, lift your arms to the sides, parallel to the ground. Palms are facing down. Hold the breath for a second or two and make a connection between the palm and the earth. Exhale slowly without moving your arms and feel the energy of the earth.

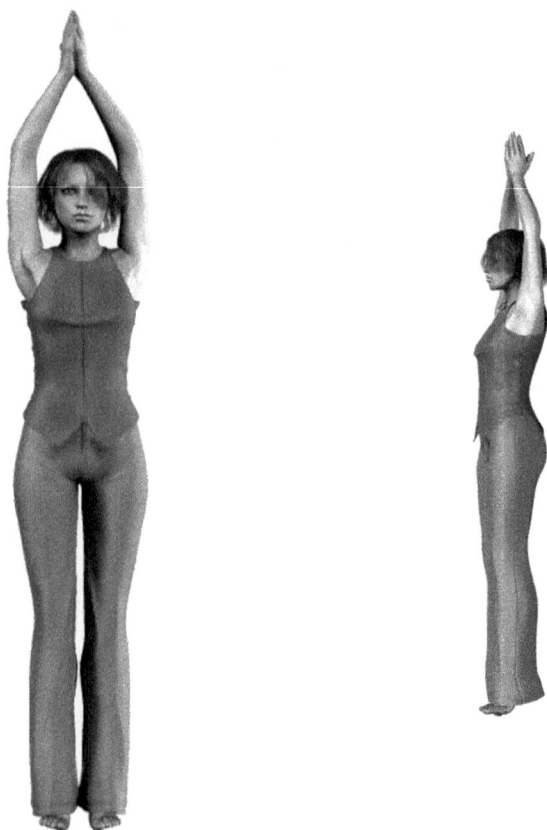

Inhale, sweeping your arms overhead, with the palms, pressing against each other. Hold you breath for a few seconds, as
you stretch up, balancing on your toes. Elongate the spine.
Focus on the tension in your palms, and tighten every muscle
of the body.
Exhale slowly, and lower your arms, relaxing your muscles.
Feel the energy rushing into your arms and shoulders, and
the opening of the chest and lungs.

Repeat two more times.

[57]

Energization Exercise #2

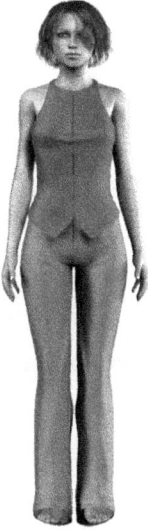

The first two postures of this exercise are the same as those from Energization Exercise #1

Stand firmly but relaxed and feel the body and the breath as instructed in the previous exercise.

Inhale slowly through the nostrils. Lift your arms to the sides. Palms are facing down. Hold the breath for a second or two and make a connection between the palm and the earth. Exhale slowly without moving your arms and feel the energy of the earth.

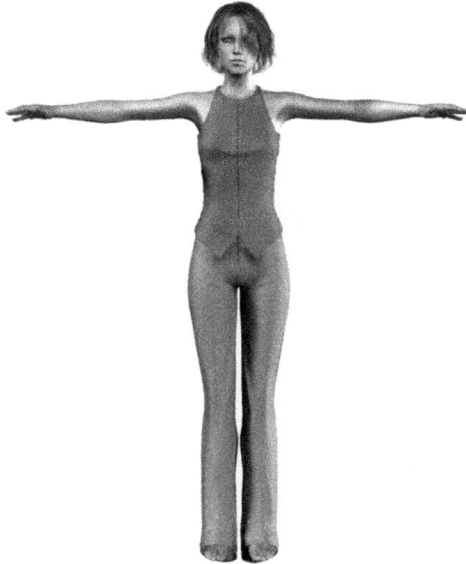

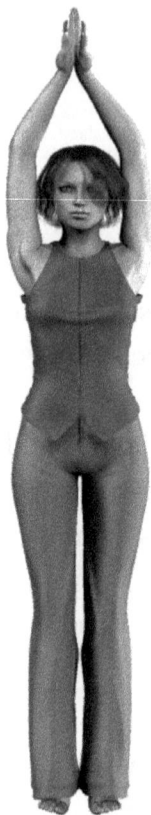

Inhale, sweeping your arms overhead, with the back of the palms, pressing against each other. Hold you breath for a few seconds, as you stretch up, balancing on your toes. Elongate the spine. Focus on the tension in your palms, and tighten every muscle of the body.

Exhale slowly, and lower your arms, relaxing your muscles. Feel the energy rushing into the back of the arms and the area around the shoulder-blades.

Repeat two more times.

Relax with feet together and arms by the side.

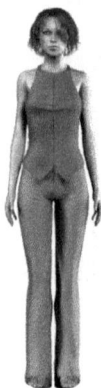

Energization Exercise #3

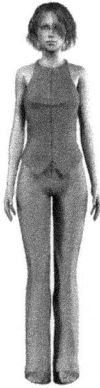

Stand straight with hands by your side. Eyes are softly focused ahead. Become aware of the body. Become aware of the air passing through your nostrils. Feel your feet sink into the floor.

Spread your feet shoulder-width apart. Arms are by the side. Eyes are focused on the tip of the nose. Palms are facing outward. Become aware of the breath, and the palms.

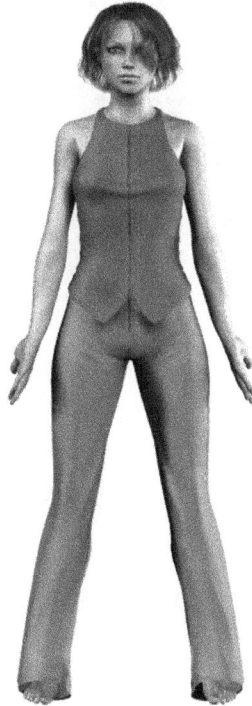

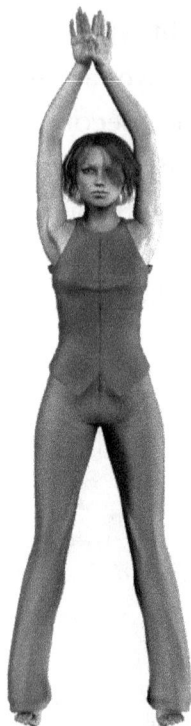

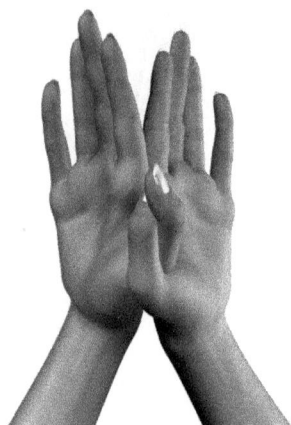

Inhale, stretching arms up, and overhead. Lock the thumbs together, with the left thumb on top of the right, pulling one thumb against the other, to create tension. Balance on the tips of your toes.

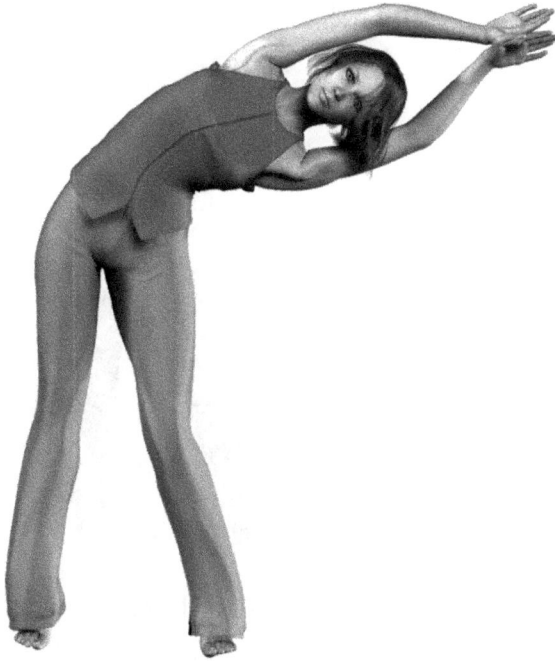

Exhale, and bend slowly to the left side, keeping
the elbows in line with the ears. Hold the breath
out for a few seconds, as you feel the tension
along the right side of the body, from the right
toes, to the right thumb.

Inhale and return to the upright position, keeping
arms overhead, and thumbs interlocked. Repeat
the left-bend two more times, and then relax arms
to the sides. Become aware of the movement of
the energy, during the relaxation.

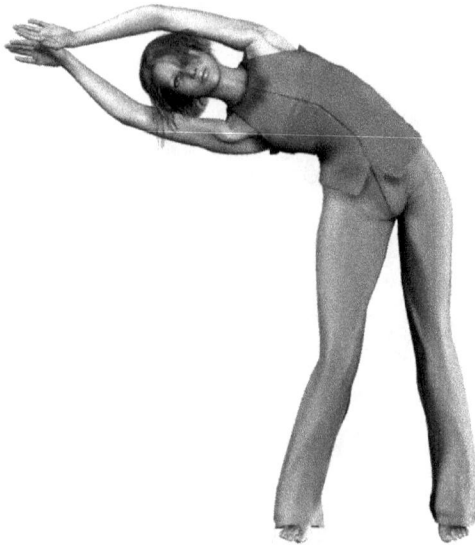

Inhale, stretching arms overhead. Lock
the thumbs, with the right thumb on top
of the left, pulling one thumb against
the other, to create tension.Exhale, and
bend slowly to the right side, keeping
the elbows in line with the ears. Hold
the breath out for a few seconds, as you
feel the tension along the left side of
the body, from the left toes, to the left
thumb. Inhale and return to the upright
position, Repeat the right-bend two
more times, and then relax arms to the
sides. Become aware of the movement
of the energy, during the relaxation.

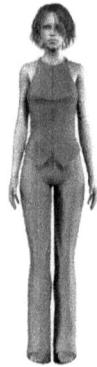

Energization Exercise #4

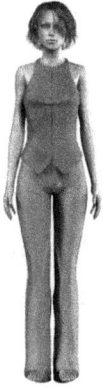

Stand straight with hands by your side. Eyes are softly focused ahead. Become aware of the body. Become aware of the air passing through your nostrils. Feel your feet sink into the floor.

Focus your eyes just above the ridge of the nose, between the eyebrows. Clasp your thumbs behind your back, with the left thumb on top of the right.

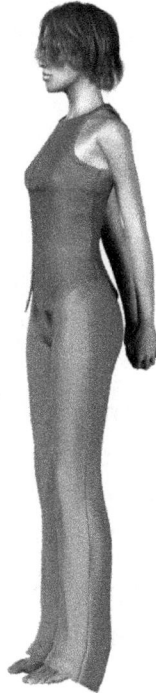

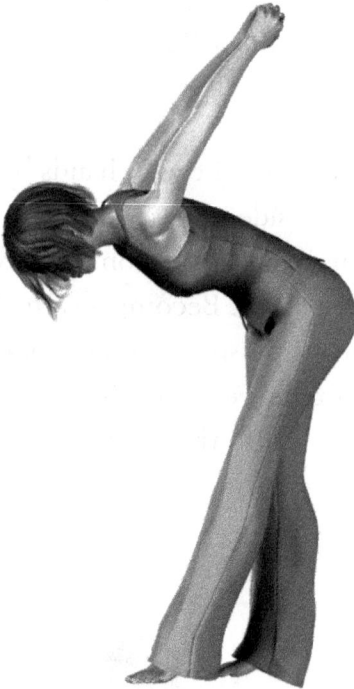

Inhale, and step forward
with the left foot. Ex-
hale, and bend forward.
lifting your arms as high
as possible. Slowly, lift
the chin up, to feel the
tension in the throat,
and lower abdomen.
Hold this position, with
the breath out, for a few
moments.

Inhale and return to the upright
position. Relax, but keep the
thumbs together.

Repeat the movement two more
times, and then return to the
beginning stance.

Relax completely, feeling the
movemnt of energy.

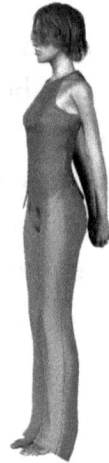

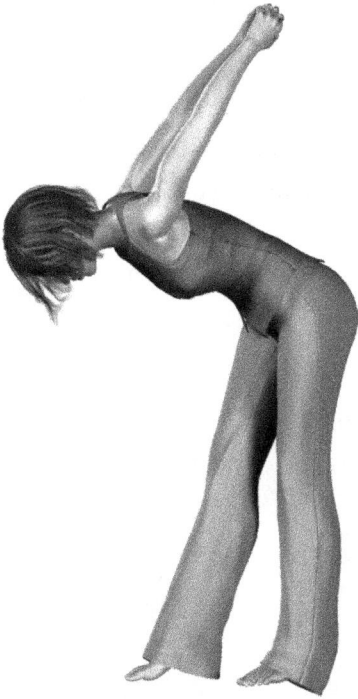

Clasp your thumbs behind your back, this time, with the right one on top.

Step out with the right leg, on the inhalation. Bend forward with the exhalation, and lifting your arms as high as possible. Slowly, lift the chin up, to feel the tension in the throat, and lower abdomen. Hold this position, with the breath out, for a few moments before returning to upright position,

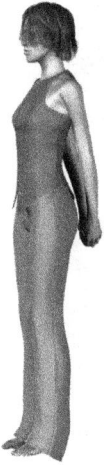

Repeat movement for 2 more times and then ruturn to staring positions.

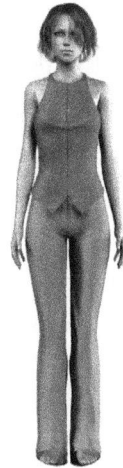

Completely relax, and become aware of the flow of energy.

Energization Exercise #5

Stand straight with hands by your side, and feet together. Eyes are softly focused ahead. Become aware of the body. Become aware of the air passing through your nostrils. Feel your feet sink into the floor.

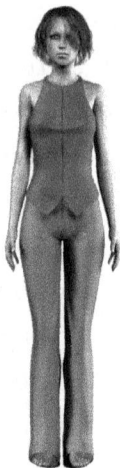

As you start your inhalation, bring your palms together at the heart level, pressing them together.

Continue to raise the arms overhead.

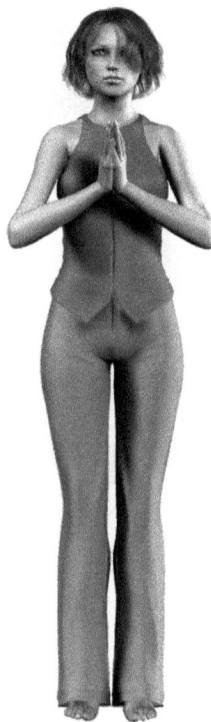

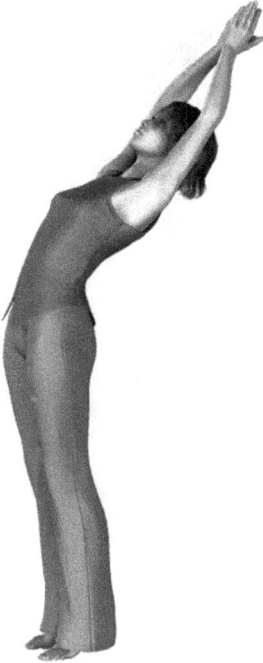

Lean back
slowly, while
holding the
breath, dropping
the head back.
Arch the back
carefully, main-
taining tension
in the arms.

Focus on the
sacrum, as you
tense the hold
body, for a few
moments.

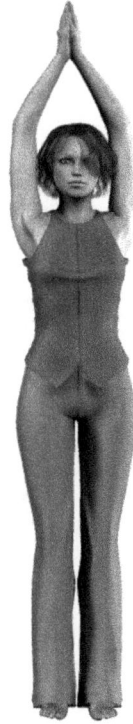

Exhale slowly, releasing all tension, passing through the
upright position, and bending forward. The arms are
parallel to the ground. Feel the stretch in the arms and
spine, accompanied by the movement of energy.

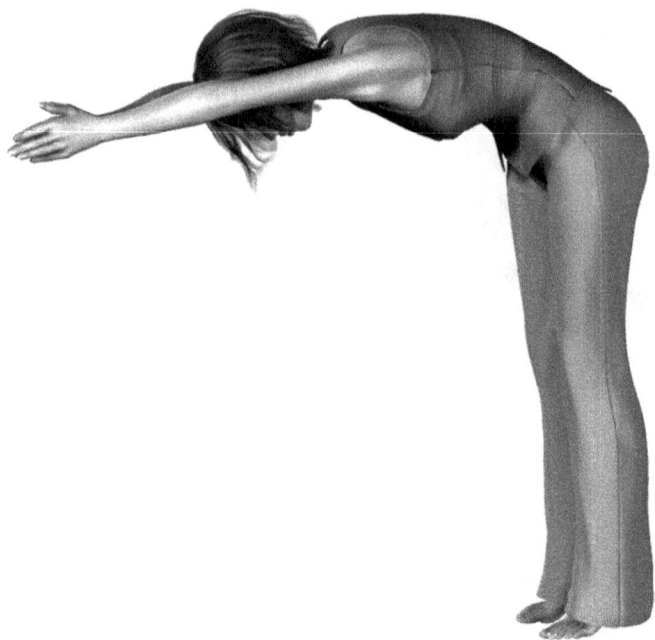

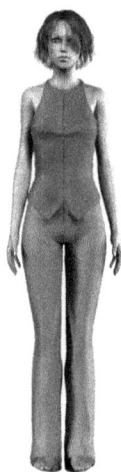

Inhale and Return to the starting position. Repeat two more times.

Then release your arms to your sides, and completely relax.

Energization Exercise #6

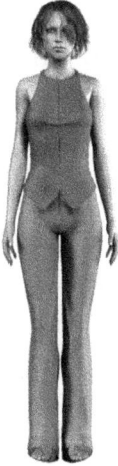

Stand straight with hands by your side, and feet together. Eyes are softly focused ahead. Become aware of the body. Become aware of the air passing through your nostrils. Feel your feet sink into the floor. Focus your awareness at the navel.

Inhale and press the arms against the sides of the body.

As you begin exhalation, relax the tension, and swing the right arm up to eye-level, bending the elbow. At the same time, swing the left arm to the left back-side, bending the left elbow. Swing from the waist, to the left, as far as comfortable. Hold the breath out in this position, for a few moments only. Then return to the first position, with the inhalation.
Repeat two more times.

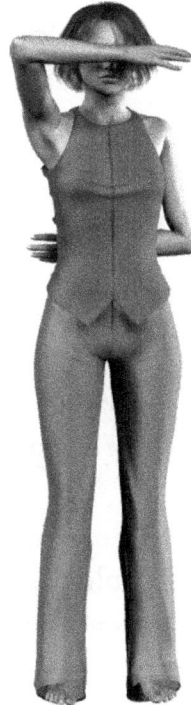

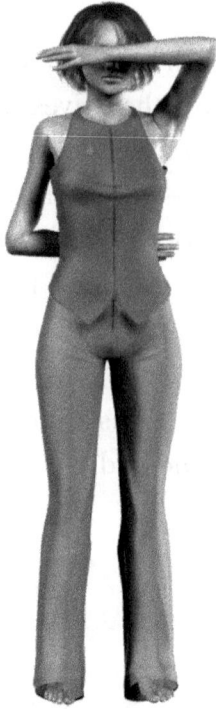

Begin exhalation, and swing the left arm up to eye-level, bending the elbow. Simulataneously, swing the right arm to the lower back. Swing to the right, from the waist. Hold the breath out, in this position, for a few seconds. Then inhale back to the starting position. Repeat two more times.

Return to starting position. Inhale and press the arms against the sides of the body.

Exhale slowly and relax completely, feeling the energy in your body.

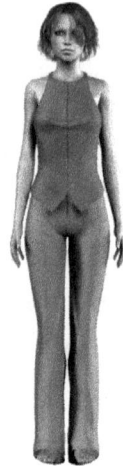

Part 3

Longevity & Health
with
Prana Energy

In Parts 1 and 2, we have shown how breath is the main support for life. We have also explained why training in the breath is the essential method for achieving physical health and a strong vibrant body filled with energy. We also hinted that said that through training in prana energy we can heal and release all physical and mental problems completely. Ultimately, this is the experience of the Eastern traditions.

We are now ready to explore beyond the physical body that we are familiar with and touch upon our subtle body and the hidden parts of our subtle physiology which provide keys to our true health and longevity.

In the yogic teachings, it is said that all human beings wish for happiness, but among all those beings who are wishing for happiness, it is extremely rare to meet a person who actually knows how to find it. Working with prana energy gives us the opportunity to find authentic happiness day and night.

> *Relying on the physical body is not sufficient to attain true health and longevity*

From the point of view of the Yogic scriptures, an ordinary healthy person takes about 21,600 breaths in a twenty-four-hour period. Western medicine also says that the average number of breaths per day is around 21,000. If we practice awareness and training in the breath, we have an incredible number of opportunities to balance the body and mind every day. When we recognize the opportunity that training in the breath provides, we give ourselves a gift: the opportunity to transcend ordinary suffering.

Working with the breath provides us with a unique opportunity for healing because the breath is something that is with us every moment of time. It doesn't matter whether we are awake or asleep, working or sitting, lying down or even doing something active - the opportunity to train in and be aware of the breath is always with us.

In mystical traditions, not only spiritual realization but sought after accomplishments such as perpetual youth and extreme longevity arise from training in prana energy. From the point of view of Ayurveda [India Medical Tradition], if we train diligently in the prana energy until our practice becomes stable and we learn how to calm and purify any agitation that arises, we can lessen the symptoms of physical illness, and our lifespan will naturally increase. Also, because we are healthy both inside and out, the color and appearance of our complexion can become youthful and glowing. When we are mentally and emotionally balanced and healthy, it shows.

Usually, when we think about how to make ourselves happy, we seek something on the outside, an external object or event. We look for something that we think will complete us; "If only I had this, I would feel better." But when we train in prana energy, we do not need to look for anything outside of us. We do not need to go to the store and buy anything to make ourselves feel less empty, lacking, or unhappy. We do not need to turn on our notebooks, cell-phones, or video games to distract us from how we feel, because we are able to influence our own sense of physical, emotional, and spiritual balance at any moment by working with the breath. The breath is something that is readily available to us simply because we are human beings. Isn't that great!

What does it mean to gain stability in prana energy training? Someone who has achieved stable and balanced prana energy is someone who has a steadfast and even-tempered mental state. Although steady, that person is not stubborn. They are mentally flexible, patient, and not easily disturbed or agitated—like a large body of water without a lot of movement on the surface. Not only would that person's mental state be controlled and balanced but they would also be calm, relaxed, and healthy.

When the prana energy is unbalanced, we experience the tendency for worry and anxiety. Our prana energy is so consistently unstable that we have become accustomed to the feeling of instability. The moment we feel calm in the mind, our prana energy immediately becomes unbalanced again and manifests as worry and anxiety. We all know people who have this tendency, or we have this tendency ourselves: it's as if we simply need something to worry about. We may think to ourselves, "I don't have any reason to be worried about this," but we find we are unable to stop. The reason we are unable to stop these mental patterns is that we have become comfortable with, and in some cases addicted to, the feeling of unstable prana energy. At times, we can feel frightened or hesitant to go beyond our ordinary mode of being, to become balanced and healthy.

It is obvious from our discussions so far that training in prana energy and attempting to balance the elements within the physical body is not something that only yogis should focus on. Western science and Yogic philosophy agree that calm, relaxed breathing makes us healthier. Because the breath is such an excellent and abundant support for life and vitality for every being on the planet, everyone can benefit from training in the breath, working with the inhalation and exhalation.

> *Prana Energy Training Is Not Just For Yogis, it is for everyone.*
>
> *It can increase our lifespan, eliminate illness and balance the mind and emotions.*
>
> *It is a recipe for happiness*

One of the positive effects of prana energy training is that the number of times we need to breathe in one day lessens. We may notice this when we sit down to relax and become aware of the breath - there will be gaps of time where we do not need to breathe. In the case of accomplished or realized practitioners who have trained in breath practice, the number of breaths taken in one hour can become very few. The result of such practice is clarity and peace of mind, and unshakable physical health

Western medicine tells us that ill people need to breathe more often than healthy ones. However, this does not explain why breathing less often also benefits our mental and emotional health. An analogy might help. Just as when a gust of wind blows over the ocean, ripples and waves cause movement and agitation on the water's surface. When the air is calm, so is the surface of the water. It is just so with the mind. The more often we breathe, the more agitated the energy of body and mind becomes. By breathing less frequently, we begin to achieve elemental harmony. This is exactly how it is, in the case of a great yogi - as the number of breaths in a minute, an hour, a day begins to lessen, the prana energy becomes increasingly stable and balanced. Feelings of extreme mental suffering become less and less over time, so much so that the potential exists for these feelings to completely disappear.

It has been shown that regardless of the school of breath/prana training, the common factor is the self-healing of the body and mind and the achievement of longevity. A person's qualities of physical and mental well-being are directly connected to prana energy training. When we can maintain a state of calm and relaxation in body, speech, and mind, we are able to accomplish more in our lives and for the betterment of society. We make clear and thoughtful decisions and have more harmonious relationships. We avoid doing things that are at odds with our personal goals and integrity, and do not sabotage our own growth. We avoid making impulsive decisions, or speaking impulsive words, ones we may regret later. When we are balanced on the inside, the world outside reflects our sense of inner harmony. If we train in prana energy, each of us has the ability both to discover a more joyful life here and now and, ultimately, to cultivate wisdom.

The Subtle Body System

In order to progress in prana energy training, we need to expand our knowledge horizon beyond what is familiar. The physical body is what most of us identify with. It is the only reality which the majority of humanity recognizes, being composed of blood and bones, the nervous system and sense organs. However, as we progress with our breath/prana training, we begin to become aware of sublter dimensions of our being. The sages have discovered the hidden physiology of multidimensional being and have taught us to consider ourselves to have five overlapping bodies or 4 coverings to our physical body. [Refer figure 15]

The energy body is just above our normal conscious perception, but can be sensed in recognition of the presence of vitality. It is like an overlay on the physical body energizing and regulating the physical cells. It acts as a channel between the physical world and the higher subtle worlds. Here is where the chakras or energy centers are particularly active. Here is also the main focus of the practice of prana energy training. This energy body is also called the pranayamakosha.

The emotional body serves as the mediation between the physical and mental bodies, converting the physical vibrations from the neutral sensations into the "emotionally charged sensations" by adding the qualities of "pleasant" or "unpleasant" or encapsulating it with feelings such as desire or fear. Most physical diseases arise from the emotional or energy bodies.

The mental body is the abode of knowledge and analytical thinking. The "emotionally charged sensations" from the emotional body is processed into perceptual units and fitted into patterns calling forth responses which vibrate back through the emotional body back into the physical realm, causing a physical reaction. This is the realm of thoughts and habit patterns.

The causal body is both the home of wisdom and of our *karmic* debts. This is the abode of the evolving soul. Higher abstract and intuitive insights arise from here.

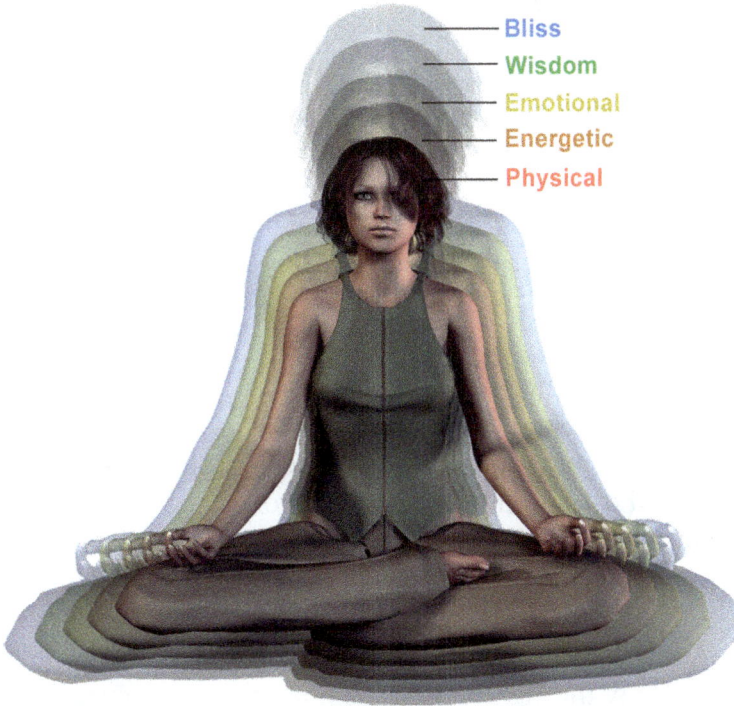

Bliss
Wisdom
Emotional
Energetic
Physical

Figure 15:
The Five Body Model For Prana Energy Training

Although for the purpose of Prana Energy training, we are going to be focusing on the Energy Body, it is important to understand that the other four bodies rely on the prana to function - our emotions and thoughts are fueled by prana, just as electricty is necessary for any electronic device.

The five-body complex exists and functions in different 'dimensions' and each is maintained by a different type of energy, from the physical chemical reactions to the subtlest consciousness energy. Each of the bodies has its own energy centers or *chakras* as well as energy channels for controlling and distributing their own level of energy. Orthodox science only recognizes the centers and channels associated with the physical body, where the cardio-vascular system represents the channels, and the brain and various nerve plexuses correspond to the energy centers. As the *chakras* are activated and awakened, you will become aware of the corresponding dimension of reality, giving you a fuller understanding of the lower dimensions.

The *Chakras or energy centers*

We will know examine in more detail the anatomy of the energy body. It has been pointed out in ancient yogic texts, that yogis are those who truly know the chakras or Energy Centers. This exemplifies how critical and potentially complex this whole topic can become.

These Energy Centers cannot be found by dissecting the physical body, but only through achieving higher states of consciousness. Figure 16 gives the location of the chakras in relation to the physical body. These energy centers are called wheels because of the circular movement of the energies that whirl in and out of them. They are also visualized as lotuses in ancient texts for the purpose of certain healing and meditation exercices.

These Energy Centers are affected by changes in our internal states, as well as by external vibrations, such as thoughts, words, or actions of others. In the average person, these centers are functioning sub-optimally, and are not harmonized with each other. As the health of the person is decreased through pollution and tension, the more out of tune these centers become. These energy centers store, convert and distribute the prana energy. They are linked to each other and to the the whole energy body by a network of energy channels called nadis which we will examine in the next section.

There are countless energy centers but the major seven are:

Center 1 [*Muladhara*]: This is also called the Root Center, and is located at the base of the spine in the perineum and is the root and support of all the other centers. It is connected with the subtle element "earth" representing solidity, and therefore is closely related to the physical body. It controls the health of the bones and structural parts of the physical body.

Center 2 [*Swadhisthana*]: This is located two inches above the 1st Center along the spine, and is associated with the subtle element water, representing fluidity and movement. This is the center for the emotional body. It is important for the health of the reproductive system.

Center 3 [*Manipura*]: This is located at the level of the navel, and is associated with the subtle element fire, representing transformation of energy. This center is closely related to the energy body. It also controls the digestive system in the physical body.

Center 4 [*Anahata*]: This is located at the spine at the heart level and is associated with the subtle element air, representing the mind and is the center for connecting with the the mental body. It is controlling the prana energy for the physical heart and circulatory system.

Center 5 [*Vishuddhi*]: This is located at the throat and is associated with the subtle element ether, representing consciousness. This is the center for the causal or spiritual body, and is considered the seat of the higher soul. This center also controls the hormonal system in the body as well as the organs of speech and the immune system.

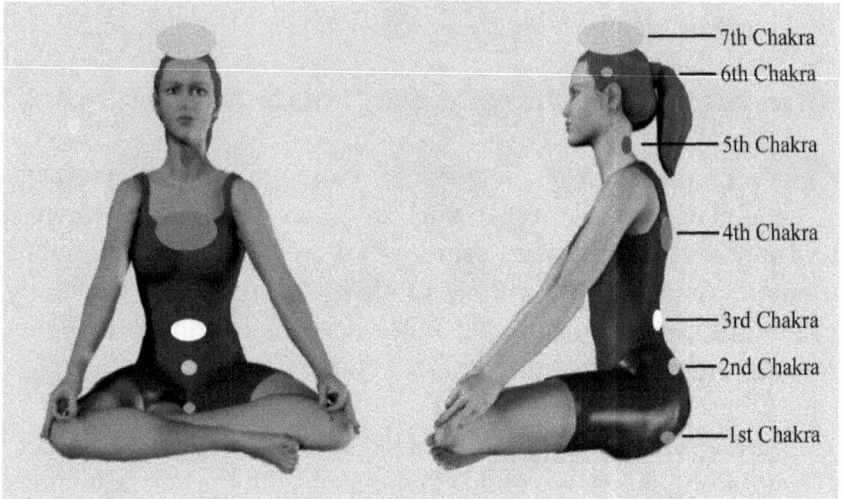

Figure 16:
Location of the Energy Centers (Chakras)

Center 6 [*Ajna*]: This is located in the center of the head at the level just above the eyes, traditionally called the "third eye" and is the center for superconsciousness. It controls the health of the physical brain and the nervous system.

Center 7 [*Sahasrara*]: This is located at the crown of the head and is associated with the Absolute or Transcendent Reality. It has not relationship to the health of the body.

We will be working on these energy centers indirectly. We have already started working on them with the previous exercises in Part 1 and Part 2. For more direct energy center techniques, you can consult my book: *Chakra self-Healing by the Power of Om.*

The Nadis - the energy channels

The nadis are a network of energy channels situated throughout the pranamayakosha [Energy Body]. The two primary nourishing energy channels are the ida and the pingala. The ida and the pingala are situated on the left and right sides of the physical spinal cord. The vital life-force, prana energy, flows through these energy channels or tubes. In between these two channels is the sushumna nadi, which is the spiritually significant of all the energy tubes. The sushumna nadi is the central channel into which the yogi tries to direct the prana to flow, so as to stimulate and awaken the kundalini, or primordial potential energy for self-realization.

For our purposes in this book, we will be focusing our attention on the left and right channels because these are the ones that are important for our health and longevity. These two subtle energy channels can be accessed physically by focusing on the left and right sides of the body and on the left and right nostrils where they have their ending position.

The scientists of prana found that during the course of a day, the flow of air or prana is flowing more in either the ida nadi (left nostril) or the pingala nadi (right nostril), or evenly flowing through the sushumna nadi (both nostrils). You can test this for yourself by moistening the back of the hand and breathing on it, to feel in which nostril the air is flowing more predominantly, or block one of the nostrils at a time and breathing through the other. You will find that the flow of air through the nostrils is very rarely equal.

Under normal circumstances, when the breath and the nadis are functioning normally, the breath flow alternates between the left and the right nostril. Modern scientists have confirmed this phenomenon, but have not discovered either the cause or purpose of this alternating breath flow, aside from speculating that it may help to regulate the body's temperature. Prana yogis have through their insight, claimed that the alternation of the natural breath flow in each nostril is due to biological changes caused by the mind's fluctuating mental states, as well as to environmental and lunar influences.

A few of the observations from the scientists of Prana Energy training concerning this phenomena, in relation to the moon, are given, just to demonstrate the depth and thoroughness of these yogic scientists:

- The ida nadi is dominant at sunrise, on the first lunar day when the moon is waxing.

- The breath flow alternates between ida and pingala, at the end of each hour.

- The breath flow continues alternating every hour for three days.

- On the fourth day at sunrise the pingala nadi becomes dominant.

- On the first lunar day, when the moon is waning, there is breath reversal at sunrise, and pingala nadi becomes dominant.

Right now, you might be wondering why these *yogis* spent so much time observing the flow of breath. **It's because they found the significant fact that a person's mental state would change with the change in nostril dominance**. When the breath flow is dominant in the right nostril a person is more inclined to physical action than to thinking or intellectual pursuits. This is because the right nostril is associated with the solar current, warmth, heat, action and the physical. It is also associated with left brain activities, such as analytic, logical and linear thinking.

When the left nostril is dominant, the mental state becomes peaceful, calm, almost dreamy. The cool moon current influences the right brain tendencies of introspection, mental creativity and higher intuition.

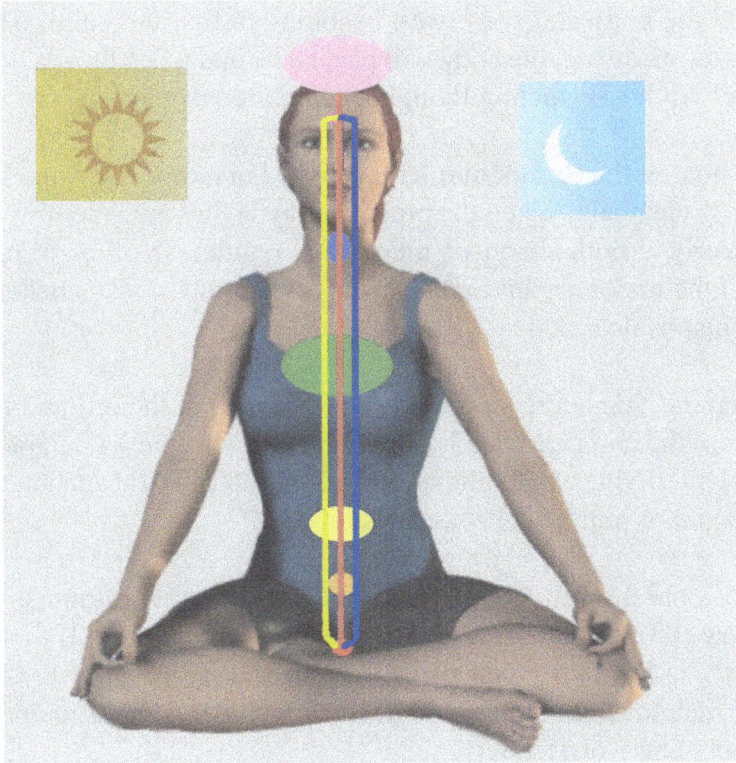

Figure 17:
The left [Moon - Ida] and right [Sun - Pingala] energy channels

It has also been found that this natural rhythm changes with our fluctuating mental and emotional states, activities, disease, stress and the unbalancing of our daily routines. This natural rhythmic cycle is necessary for balancing the mind and body. There would be an imbalance, and serious harm can occur, if the breath were to flow in only one nostril for 24 hours or more, an indication of serious illness.

When the breath is flowing equally through both nostrils, then the sushumna nadi is active and successful meditation is possible. In this balanced state, the mental processes become clear and calm while the body and the breath becomes steady and calm. If the pingala is flowing, the body will be restless and when the ida flows, there will be distracting thoughts and a dreamy state.

The goal of the **Sun-Moon Breath** is to balance the left and right energy channels. When the prana energy is flowing smoothly and regularly in both channels, then it will regulate the flow of prana to all the major organs and systems of the body. This is benefical for the physical body.

When the Sun and Moon breaths are balanced, the left and right sides of the brain are equally active and this will enables heightened problem solving capabilities - a marriage of the logical and intuitive potential of human consciousness.

Emotional stability is achieved because of the calmness and increased self-awareness that results from the balance. If the Sun energy is to much, then there is restlessness, inability to focus and rush to anger, while too much Moon energy leads to apathy, anxiety and worries.

Guidelines for the Practice of Prana Energy Training

Place

Select a peaceful, clean, warm, airy place where you can sit without disturbance by noise, family members, or visitors. It can be a special room, or a dedicated part of a room, or even a garden.

Time

Traditionally, it is recommended that Prana Energy training be best started in spring or during the waxing phase of the moon. However, if you need to start the training, anytime is a good time. It can be practiced throughout the year, but do not practice in the heat of the sun or when the body is cold or ill. Just before or during sunrise and after sunset are excellent times for practice.

Posture

The posture you sit in should allow you to keep your back erect from the base of the spine to the neck and you should be able to sit comfortably and relaxed with your eyes closed.

A folded blanket or cushion can be used to lessen the strain. In the next section, are described the recommended postures: sukhasana (easy pose), siddhasana (perfected pose), padmasana (lotus pose) and vajarasan (kneeling pose). These postures all require being able to bend the knees. If you have a knee problem or it is too painful, then it's best to sit on the edge of chair.

Precautions

Do not practice Prana Energy training immediately after meals. Wait at least two hours after eating. If you are hungry, just eat a small snack or drink some liquid. You can eat fifteen minutes after the practice.

Do not force or strain the breath. Avoid jerky movements. Do not struggle to restrain the breath after inhalation or exhalation. If you feel any negative effects, then stop your practice immediately and rest. Use your common sense.

Start out by practicing for no more than twenty minutes, to ensure there is no strain and fatigue. One of the goals of the training is to increase energy, and decrease stress. Slowly, over months, you may extend the time to one hour, or more.

Be regular in your practice. It is more beneficial to practice a little everyday, than it is to practice a lot for a few days and then stop for a few days, before resuming.

Postures for Prana Energy Training

Unless otherwise instructed in the exercises themselves, there are four postures recommended for comfortable and stable sitting – they are *sukhasana, siddhasana, padmasana,* and *vajrasana.* The choice is based on your individual preference and capability.

The physical discipline of sitting correctly is itself of great benefit for the energy system, as well as enhancing mental discipline and improving the powers of concentration.

The four postures that can be used, as shown in figures 18 and 19 and 20:

1. *Sukhasana* or 'easy pose' is a cross-legged posture that is the customary relaxed sitting posture on the floor. You may wish to sit on a cushion so as to elevate your pelvis above your legs to decrease the pressure on the legs.

2. *Siddhasana* or 'perfect pose' is the yogic meditation posture that is highly recommended for increasing the flow of prana. Sit with your legs stretched forward. Bend your left leg and place the heel of the left foot against the perineum.Bend your right leg over the left and place it on the left thigh with the right heel resting against the pubic area. The knees should be touching the floor. For ladies, it

is not necessary to place a leg against the pubic areas. It is sufficient to place it on the floor close to the left leg. Also, it is advisable to exchange the left and right leg positions if the knees cause a problem.

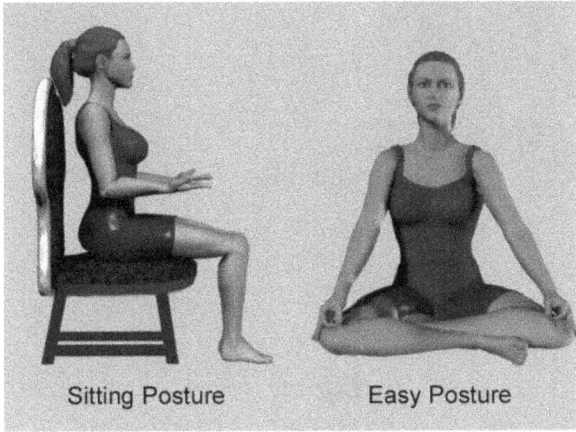

Figure 18:
Chair Position and Easy Posture

3. *Padmasana* or the 'lotus posture' has great benefits, if you can get into it without too much strain. Extend both legs forward and bend your right leg carefully over the left, placing it on the left thigh, as close to the groin as possible. Bend your left leg at the knee and place the left foot on the right thigh. It will take some practice to be able to get into and stay in this posture comfortably. A modified and simpler posture is called the half-lotus, where the left leg is simply tucked in under the right. It is also good to exhange the right and left leg positions so as to balance the knees.

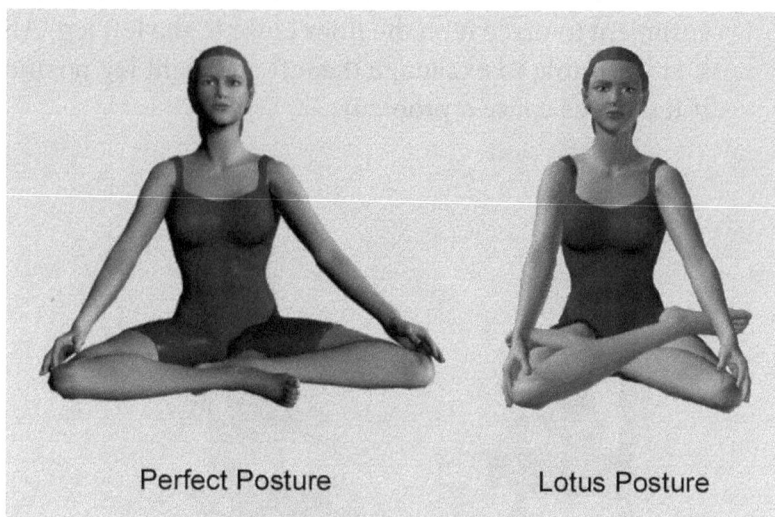

Perfect Posture   Lotus Posture

Figure 19:
Perfect Pose and Lotus Posture

4. *Vajrasana* or 'kneeling pose'. Sit in a kneeling position, with head, neck and trunk straight. It is also possible to put a cushion or stool between the seat and the legs, to reduce the pressure on the feet.

Another consideration during the practice is the position of the hands and arms. There are three simple positions that can be used with any of the four postures (refer figure 21):

1. Open receptive: Rest your hands on your knees with the palms facing up.
2. Place the back of your right hand on top of your left palm with the thumbs lightly touching each other.
3. Interlace your fingers together and rest them on your lap.

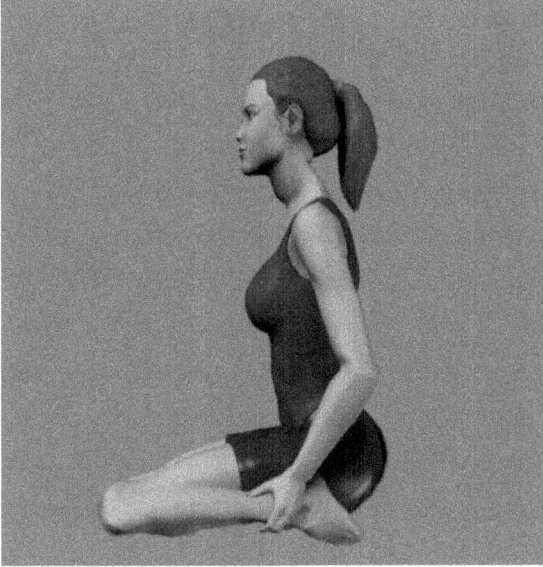

Figure 20:
Kneeling Pose

Whichever variation and combination of posture and hand position you adopt, it is important to remember not to press your arms into the body, and to relax your shoulders and chest, keeping the head and neck upright and steady.

Additional points to observe for good posture:

1. The back is straight without undue strain, so that energy can flow freely.
2. The shoulders are relaxed and not hunched forward or bent backwards.
3. The mouth should be relaxed and slightly smiling.
4. The eyes are closed but relaxed.
5. The head should be held erect without tension with the neck tucked in ever so gently.

Breathing Exercise 5: Sun-Moon Breath

A. Preparation phase

1. *Cleansing the air-passages and lungs*:
   Sit comfortably in one of the recommended postures. Place your hands on your knees. Inhale a Complete Breath. Then pucker your lips and exhale vigorously through them in a series of short, sharp exhalations as you slowly lower your trunk and forehead as close to the floor as possible. Then slowly raise your head and trunk back up while slowly breathing in through the nostrils. Perform this three times.

2. *Alternate nadi-cleansing*:
   This is especially beneficial for those suffering from sinus congestion.

   Sit in a comfortable posture with your spine straight and your body relaxed.

   Slowly inhale through both nostrils, then pucker your lips and exhale all the air from your lungs with a series of dynamic exhalations, like a bellows action.

   Closing the right nostril with your right thumb, inhale gently through the left nostril. Then close your left nostril with the third finger of your right hand and exhale through your right nostril, with a series of short, sharp exhalation.

Continue with inhaling through the right nostril, and exhaling with force through the left. This completes one round. Start the cycle again with inhaling through both nostrils. Practice three rounds.

B. Purification Phase

3. *Basic Sun-Moon Purification*:
   This is the most important Prana Energy Training technique for purifying the energy channels and strengthening the nerves of the physical body. It purifies the blood and the brain cells, and also maintains equilibrium in the catabolic and anabolic processes in the body.

   By making the breath flow in each nostril in a balanced way, the pranic flow in the Sun and Moon channels become balanced. Under these balanced conditions, prana will flow into the central channel and the left and right brains are equally stimulated.

   Sit comfortably in one of the four recommended postures, with the head, neck and spine in a straight line. Keep a smile on your face and the body relaxed.

   Place your left hand on your left knee, relaxed, and form the right hand in nasik mudra. This is formed by folding the first two fingers towards the palm keeping the thumb and the last two fingers extended. Refer to figures 21 and 22.

First, exhale through both nostrils, and then close your right nostril with your thumb and inhale slowly and deeply through your left nostril. At the end of the inhalation, close your left nostril with your ring and little fingers, release your thumb from the right nostril and exhale through your right nostril. Next, inhale through your right nostril, then close it with your thumb and exhale through your left nostril.

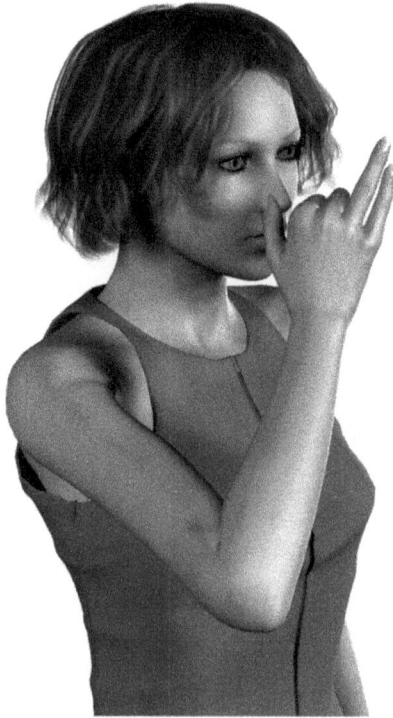

Figure 22:
Sun-Moon Breath - closing right nostril

This completes one round. Practice only 6 rounds to begin with, then gradually increase to 12 rounds after a few weeks.

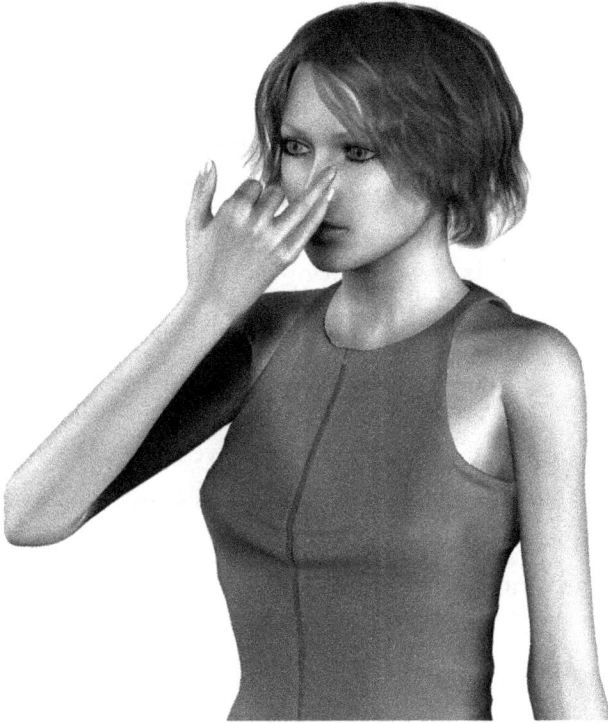

Figure 23:
Sun-Moon Breath: exhaling through the right nostril

4. *Advanced Sun-Moon Purification*:
   Add this part to your Prana Energy Training only after you have practiced the Basic technique for at least one month. This uses the same alternating breathing pattern

as in the Basic Sun-Moon Breath, adding the counting of the length of inhalation and exhalation, which was learned in Calming Breath [Part 1].

In the Calming Breath, we learnt to inhale and exhale to the same count. The relative ratios of breath inhalation, retention) and exhalation) are: 1:0:1:0 This means that there is no breath retention and that the exhalation is the same as that of the inhalation. For the Advanced Sun-Moon Breath, we use a ratio of 1:0:2:0, that is, the exhalation is twice as long as the inhalation. There is no holding of breath between inhalation and exhalation.

Begin with a minimum inhalation count of six and therefore an exhalation of twelve for the first week. Do not increase the count until you can practice this with comfort and ease, and then increase the count to 8 for inhale and 16 for exhale.

First, practice three rounds of inhaling and exhaling through the left nostril with the required ratio. Then perform three rounds of inhaling and exhaling through the right nostril with the same ratio. This helps to setup the rhythym of the breath.

Continue with the alternating or Sun-Moon breath. Apply nasik mudra, and inhale through the left nostril, counting the length of the inhalation. Exhale through the right nostril, making the exhalation twice as long as the inhalation. Breathe in through the right nostril, counting the length of the inhalation, and then exhale through the left nostril, making the exhalation twice as long as the inhalation. This is one round. Continue for a total of six rounds.

Caution on the holding of breath

There is a lot of misunderstanding about the practice of breath retention or holding of breath during Prana Energy Training . This is due to the popularization of advanced *Yogic* texts, which appear to promote this practice indiscriminately. In general, holding of breath can put a stress on your heart and circulatory system, elevating the blood pressure several times above normal, which can result in ruptured blood vessels or a stroke.

What may not be clear from books is that beginners in *Yoga* are not taught the holding of breath, until they have had years of practice in strengthening the body, circulatory system and nervous systems, and only after authorization and personal supervision from their teachers. When holding of breath is taught, it should always be accompanied by the practice of the muscular locks or bandhas. The holding of breath is not necessary or even recommended for the therapeutic purpose of Prana Energy Training. It is an important aspect of the mystical side of breath practice for attaining higher states of consciousness.

It is my personal experience and observation, that most breathing techniques do not require the active and forced breath retention, but will over time, increase the natural pause between the inhaled breath and the exhaled breath. This natural pause does not put a strain on the heart.

Ayurveda and pranic healing

According to the ancient health science of India, called Ayurveda, all forms of matter are made up of the combination and condensation of the five Cosmic Elements of Space,(or Ether), Air, Fire, Water, and Earth. Although all material things are constituted from all five elements, they are differentiated according to the proportion of each element.

This knowledge is applied to the human body and constitution through the system of classification, called the *doshas*. In matter where the Air Element predominates, it is described as having a vata constitution or dosha. There are three primary dosha*s* used to describe the human body. Besides vata dosha, when Fire predominates, it is called pitta, and kapha for the predominance of Water and Earth.

Every human body may be classified into one of the three *doshas*. There are a small number of people, who may be combinations of more than one dosha, for example pitta-kapha, or vata-pitta.

On one level, our physical body has all three *doshas* working together. For example, the digestive system is pitta or Fiery in nature, the nervous system is vata or Airy, while tissues are kapha or Watery. This perspective helps in understanding how yoga practice, particularly Prana Energy Training affects the various organs and systems of the body.

At a higher level, one of the doshas predominates, not only the body structure, but also tendencies towards specific types of ill-health, as well as emotional reactions. This perspective helps to understand the affects of prana practice on the three distinct body-emotion-mind types. Different foods are prescribed for the three doshas, and each has a set of 'beneficial' and 'harmful' table of foods, for attaining optimal health. Similarly, it is necessary to adapt one's lifestyle according to the body type. For example, pitta types should learn to relax more than the other types and deal with anxieties and temper tantrums - they should perform more 'cooling' energy practices, and less 'heating' energy techniques..

There are certain generalizations which are helpful to prevent ill-health: vata types are prone to mental or nervous disorders, pitta types have a tendency towards inflammations and infections, while kapha types suffer from overweight and swollen glands.

All doshic imbalances can be alleviated by proper diet, and in most cases, a balancing of the five vayus or pranas, which will be explained in the next section. There is also a set of techniques to balance the five elements that will the sevven technique we will incorporate into the Prana Energy Program [PEP].

The two most important vayus are prana and apana, and they can be balanced by the alternate nostril **Sun-Moon** breathing technique given earlier in Part three.

The Ten Vayus and the Five Vital Pranas

Once prana enters the physical body through the vehicle of the breath, it takes on certain differentiated functions and become localized near certain major parts of the body, and move intelligently as required. The differentiated pranas are called vayus (vital airs) and there are ten of them in our "energy body". The five major vayus function through the five subsidiary nerve centers in the brain and spinal cord and are the ones that we will want to balance in order to attatin well-being and longevity.

The Five Major Vayus [refer figure 24]

Udana vayu functions in the body between the larynx and the top of the head. It controls speech, the sense of balance, memory and intellect. Udana has an upward movement – it carries kundalini[the potential energy for self-realization] to the crown or seventh energy center, sahasrara. It separates the astral body and physical body at the time of death. Udana is pale white in color.

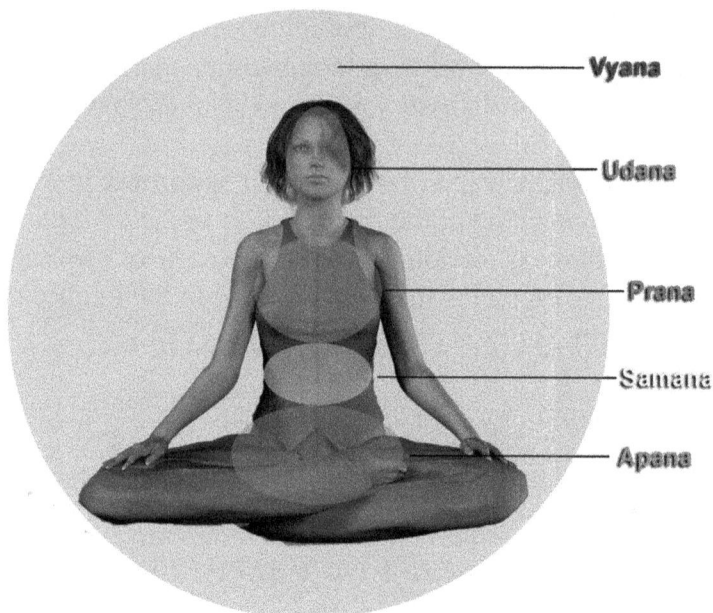

Figure 24:
The Five Pranas

Prana vayu functions in the region between the larynx and base of the heart. It controls speech, the respiratory muscles, blood circulation and body temperature. Prana is the color of coral.

Samana vayu functions between the heart and the navel region, maintaining a balance between apana and *prana*. It controls all the metabolic activity involved in digestion. Samana is translucent milky white to yellow in color.

Apana vayu functions in the region from the navel to the feet. It normally has a downward movement, but under certain circumstances will carry the kundalini upwards in Sushumna [the central nadi or energy channel coincident with the spinal cord] to unite with prana. This apana controls the functions of the kidneys, excretory system, colon, rectum and sex organs and is pink in color.

Vyana vayu permeates throughout the whole body and is an aura around the body. It helps the other vayus to function properly. Specifically, it controls both the voluntary and involuntary movements of the muscles and joints, keeps the whole body upright by generating unconscious reflexes along the spine, as well as controlling the physical nerves and the nadis or subtle astral/ energy channels. Vyana is the color of a ray of sunlight.

Breathing Exercise 6: Five-Prana Breath

The following set of Prana Energy healing techniques balances all five pranas, and is highly recommended as a disease preventive, as well as helping in the treatment of diseases. It consists of six pranic techniques, which I've personally found very beneficial, and would like to share with you. Each has a different function, and effect different parts of the pranic or Energy Body:

Since there are five pranas, or five aspects of the life-force energy in the body, there are five parts to the balancing technique. During the practice, each part is repeated a number of times, and then proceeding to the next part, in the sequence. Finally, the sequence is reversed and each part is practiced for the same number of repetitions.

This balancing breath is given as a sequence incorporating all the techniques, but each can be performed by itself, if you feel the need to balance a particular vayu, or aspect of prana, but I would recommend that you practice all five parts because you may not be the best judge of what you need.

1. Prana Vayu

Although the prana vayu is concentrated at its home in the chest area, it is generally considered to be controlled by the third eye energy center in the middle of the head.

Inhale deeply, drawing energy from above and around the head, into the third-eye center, visualizing a ball of light concentrated there.

Exhale through the third eye, spreading the life-force throughout the head, and the eyes, ears, nostrils, and the mouth. Life-force is brought in all around the head through the senses, purifying them. This completes one round.

Repeat six times for a total of seven rounds.

Benefits:
Revitalizes the brain and helps against disorders of the nervous system. It is useful as treatment for sinus problems, head colds, and headaches.

2. *Udana Vayu*

Inhale deeply through the mouth and draw the life-force into the throat center.

Exhale, chanting OM aloud in a continuous manner until the breath is completely finished, Feel the sonic vibration expanding outward and upward as you chant.

Repeat six times to complete seven rounds.

Benefits:
Increases vitality and improves self-expression.
Helpful in treatment of sore throat.

3. Vyana Vayu

Inhale deeply through the heart center, while extending your arms to the sides and opening up the chest. The life-force energy is spiraling outwards. At the end of the inhalation, visualize the life-force expanding throughout the body and limbs.

Exhale back into the heart center, visualizing all the life-force returning to the heart center, spiraling inwards.

Repeat six times for a total of seven rounds.

Benefits:
Helpful in treating diseases of circulatory problems, especially lung and heart diseases.

4. Samana Vayu

Feel the navel center, and visualize the universal life-force through its galaxies, stars and planets - it is all around you. Inhale deeply, bringing the universal life-force into the navel center, spiraling inwards.

Feel the life-force as concentrated fire at the navel at the end of the inhalation.

Exhale, spiraling outward nourishing all the cells, organs and systems of the body.

Repeat the inhale-exhale cycle seven times.

Benefits:
Helpful in treating digestive system disorders and diseases of the liver and gall-bladder.

5. *Apana Vayu*

This is best done in a standing posture. Feel the perineum and visualize the connection with the center of the earth.

Inhale deeply, drawing the life-force energy down to the root center at the perineum.

Exhale from the perineum, down through the legs and feet, into the earth. This completes on round.

Repeat six times for a total of seven rounds.

Benefits:
Helpful in treating disorders of the reproduction and the excretory systems. Also useful for healing menstrual problems and sexual dysfunctions.

After practicing the sequence from steps 1 to 5, then reverse and practice from 5 to 1. That is, start the sequence from step 5, the apana vayu and end with step 1, prana vayu.

The Five Cosmic Elements

The ancient Masters of Wisdom perceived reality directly, and have transmitted their insights on cosmic evolution through countless generations. They perceived that cosmic consciousness gave rise to Universal Energy which then manifested into the five Universal Elements –Material Building Blocks of Space, Air, Fire, Water and Earth - which became the atomic building blocks of all matter and energy, through a process of grossification.

It is important to keep in mind that the translation of the these words is imperfect and should not lead you to confuse them with their common usage. When the Masters talk about Space, they are more closely pointing out the universal force of gravitation than anything resembling "open space".

From Universal Energy, the vibration of matter called the sound of Om by the ancients, caused the appearance of Space [*Akasha*], which further materialized and created AIR [*Vayu*], and from the function of it's friction movement, AIR created the Fire [*Agni*] element. From the heat of Fire, Space dissolved and liquefied and gave birth to Water [*Apas*]. When the Water element solidified, Earth [*Prithvi*] is formed. The whole of the material Universe is formed by the combinations of these five Elements.

It should be noted that these five Elements are not visible particles, but through a process of grossification, became present in all matter and energy. They refer to the etheric, gaseous, radiant, fluid, and solid states of matter and the principles of space movement, light, cohesion, and density.

As an example, the planet Earth is formed with a greater proportion of the gross aspects of the Earth Element.

When we move from the macrocosmic view of the universe and

examine the microcosmic aspect of human beings, we have to consider the interaction of these five element in the formation of the wholistic being. The five bodies of man are formed by various proportions of these five Elements. In the physical body, the solid structures such as bones, muscles, skin and hair are derived from the Earth Element. From Water Element, all the fluids and secretions are derived, while the Fire Element rules the digestive and metabolic systems. All movement of the body is governed by Air, while cavities are the province of Space. [Refer to figure 25.]

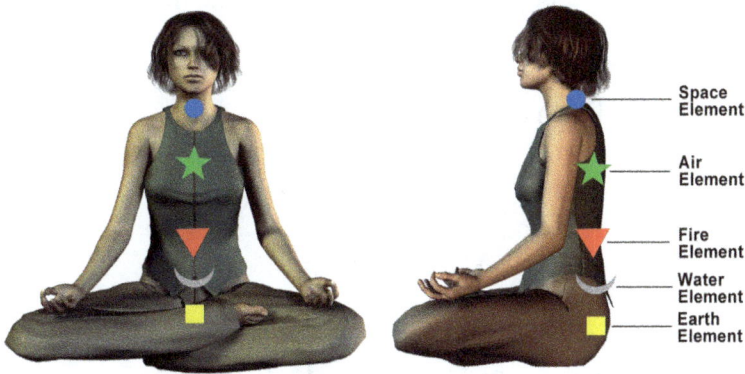

Figure 25:
The Five Elements In The Subtle Body

The five Elements also manifest in the five senses, providing for all perception of external environment. Space, Air, Fire, Water, and Earth are related to hearing, touch, vision, taste and smell respectively. Since the human body (all five bodies) are a manifestation of the five Elements, a balance of harmony of these are required for healing and health, as well as for spiritual realization.

The sages have given us techniques to observe the imbalance of the five Elements in one's physical body. It is taught that our feelings and emotions are conditioned by the particular Element which is dominating at a particular time. Therefore, by identifying the dominant Element, and observing its progression, one can gain insight into one's consciousness. By understanding this play of the Elements, the play of consciousness is penetrated, and by passing beyond the Elements, we can attain to independence from the their play on our physiological health.

According to ancient studies, the Air Element flows first, followed by Fire, Earth, Water, and Space. During a one hour period, each Element dominates for a specific time:

> Earth   : 20 minutes
> Water : 16 minutes
> Fire   : 12 minutes
> Air   : 8 minutes
> Space : 4 minutes

My favorite technique for detecting which of the five Elements is active, at a particular time in the body, is to sense the location of air passing through the nostril. This takes some sensitivity and training, but is worth the effort. There is also some differences as to the correspondence between the location and the Element.

Some texts state that when air passes through the center of the nostril, then the Earth Element is dominant, upper part is for the Fire Element, lower part for the Water Element; while when air passes obliquely, it is the Air Element, and when it is rotating, then the Space Element is present.

My own experience is that when air passes the top of the nostril, it corresponds to the Earth Element; bottom to Water; right side to Fire; left side to Air; center to Space. More research needs to be done on to identify the best way to detect the dominance of an element at any particular time in our body - this can be essential to determine the best activity or treatment for special sicknesses.

The five Elements are a composite of our bodies but there are controls centers for each of them within our energy center or chakras. Figure 26 gives the locations of those centers.

Mental and emotional imbalances, such as chronic illness or anxiety are caused by imbalances among the five elements. Harmony among the five elements in the body (air, fire, earth, water, and space) is disrupted when one element becomes disproportionately strong or weak in relation to the others. More often than not, stress, caused by a strengthening and increase of the air element, plays a tremendous role in the development of mental and emotional imbalances. In our society, anxiety and depression are the most common of these imbalances.

Everyone suffers from stress every day. When we do not know how to cope with the physical and emotional results of stress, it affects us in a profound way. Studies have shown that ninety percent of all doctor visits are related to stress, because stress exacerbates all medical conditions. Chronic stress contributes to breath related pulmonary and cardiac disorders such as heart disease, high blood pressure, and hardening of the arteries, the three health conditions that most threaten our longevity. Research also shows that stress contributes to emotional imbalances such as anxiety and depression.

Anxiety is the most common class of mental disorder worldwide, affecting millions of people. Anxiety is a broad term and includes panic disorder, generalized anxiety disorder, post-traumatic stress disorder, phobias, and separation anxiety disorder. Depression is another prevalent disorder, impacting people in all areas of the world. Depression and anxiety, both fueled by stress, are often seen together. In one study, five percent of those with major depression were also diagnosed with generalized anxiety disorder while six percent had symptoms of panic disorder. There is a lot of research that suggests some form of relationship between stress, anxiety and depression.

Even though millions of people are touched by these painful states of mind every day, understanding the imbalances of the elements in more detail may help take away the power these painful states hold over us. The good news is that through working with the breath and balancing the five elements, we actually hold the key to helping ourselves bring body and mind into balance.

No matter how out of control we feel, how low our energy is, or how large our problems seem to loom, Prana Energy training is an effective intervention for all emotional imbalances. When we work with the breath, we work with the root of the problem.

Breathing Exercise 7: Five-Element Breath

Preliminary Exercise: Connecting with the five elements

Before we begin the main portion of the Five-Element Breath, we make a connection with them and acknowledge them as the basic constituent of our bodies. The element earth is symbolized by a yellow square and represents the solid parts of the body. The bodily fluids are connected to the element of water which is in the form of a white crecent moon. The element fire is symbolized by a red triangle and is responsible for body heat and digestive system. The breath and nervous system is under the control of the air element represesented by a six-pointed green star. The space or ether element has dominion of the hollow spaces and cavities of the body - it is a blue ball.[refer figure 25]

To begin, visualize a white ball of light in front of your face. Let it expand and surround your whole body. Inhale and let the white light fill your body, exhale and let it return to the ball of light.

Next, let the ball of light become yellow in color and inhale it to your perineum. Exhale it back to the ball of light. The ball of light becomes silver in color - inhale and exhale at the site of the water element [the sacral are]. The ball of light next becomes red in color - breathe the fire element to the naval area. For the fourth breath, breathe to the air element in the back of the chest in the form of green light. Finally, conclude with the space element to the throat area in the form of blue light.

I. Balancing the Earth Element

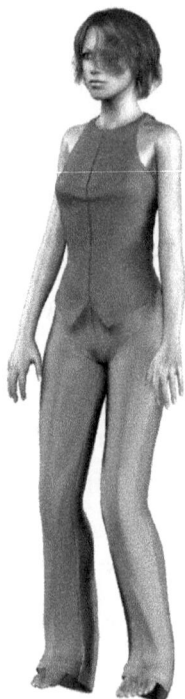

Stand with feet shoulder's width apart and hands by the sides. Relax your shoulders and tuck in the hips, aligning the back of the head with the tailbone. Feel the energy of the earth beneath your feet and on the ground around you.

Exhale and bend your upper body forward while keeping the spine straight. Let your knees bend so that you can touch the ground with your finger tips.

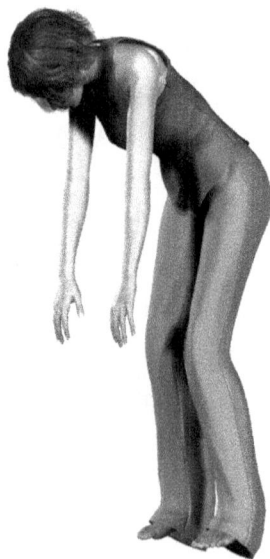

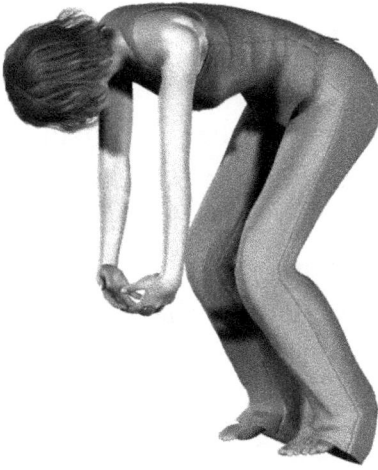

Inhale as you rise up and bring the earth energy up with your hands. Visualize yellow ball of light within your hands and arms.

Tuck in your hips and straighten you back. Knees are slightly bent. Bring the palms up simultaneously to the level of the eyes and the palms facing inwards.

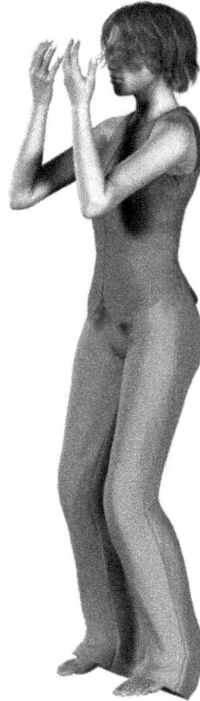

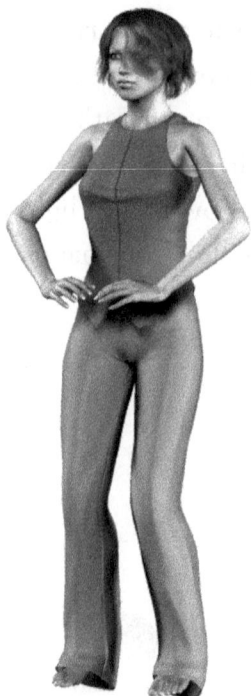

Hold the breath out for a few seconds after the exhale. Then visualize the yellow ball of light washing over your body as you turn you hands over and push down slowly to the level of the naval.

Move your hands apart and let them relax by the sides of the body. Straighten your knees. Let your-self relax and gently resume breathing.

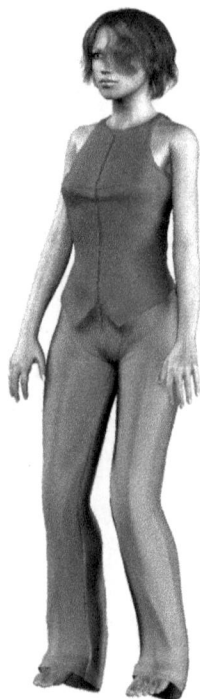

II. Balancing the Water Element

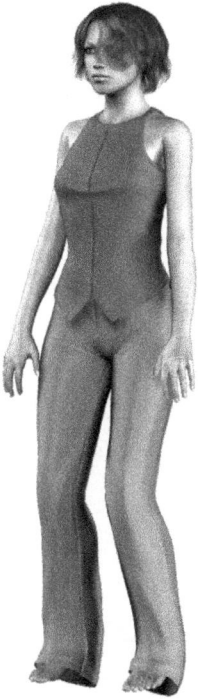

Stand with feet shoulder's
width apart and hands by the
sides. Relax your shoulders
and tuck in the hips, aligning the back of the head with
the tailbone. Feel the water
energy in your pelvic area
and visualize it as a silver light
around you.

Exhale and bend
your upper body
forward while
keeping the spine
straight. Let your
knees bend slightly
and let your head
hang loosely.

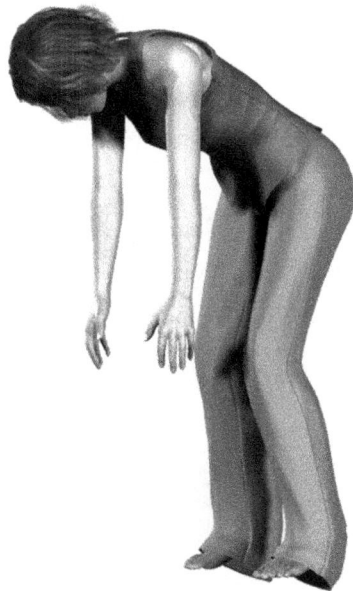

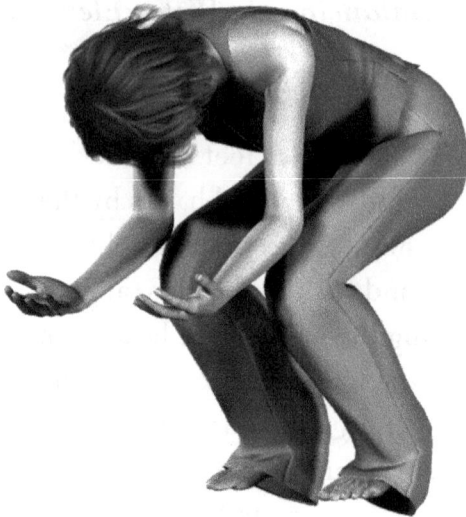

Use both hands
to form a cup
or a water ves-
sel. Dip your
hands into the
water and cup
it in your hands
as a silver light.

Inhale gently while
you straighten your
body and as you
bring your hands
with the water over
your head.

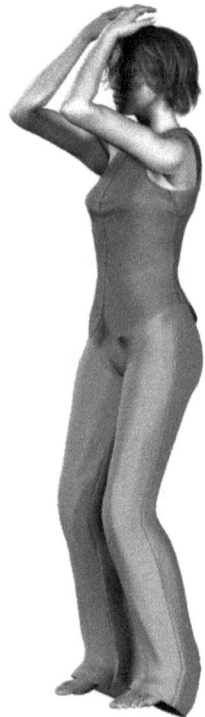

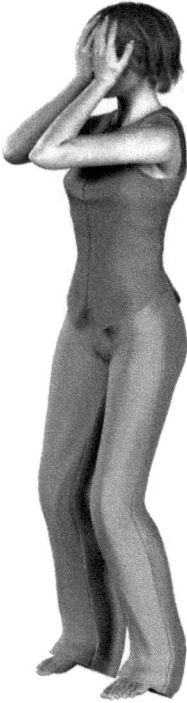

Hold your breath out for a few moments as you finish the inhale. Then, imagine the silver water running over and down your face as you exhale and rub your hands on your face.

Let your hands drop gently down to your sides and straighten your knees and tuck in your back. Relax.

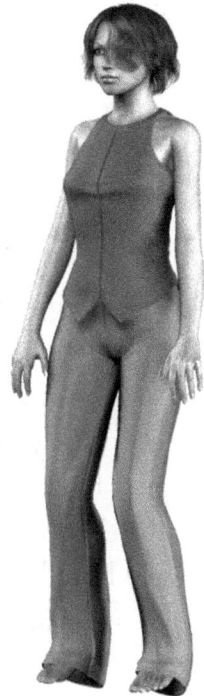

III. Balancing the Fire Element

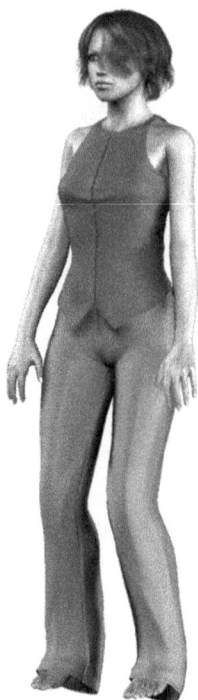

Stand with feet shoulder's width apart and hands by the sides. Relax your shoulders and tuck in the hips, aligning the back of the head with the tailbone. Exhale and bend forward as in the previous two exercise. Touch the ground with the tips of your fingers and imagine you are absorbing the heat of the fire element.

Inhale gently as you rise up and at the same time, interlock your fingers to symbolize fire. Vizualize the red light between your hands

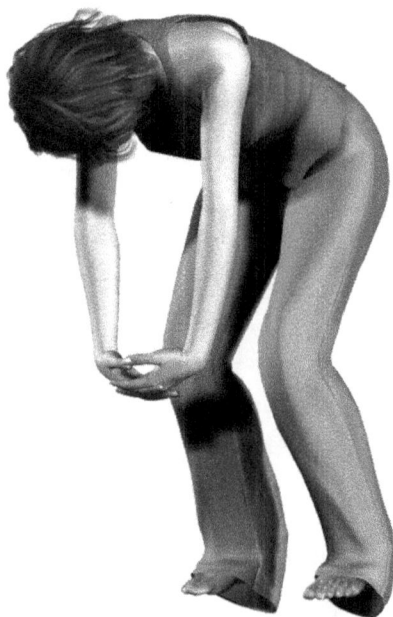

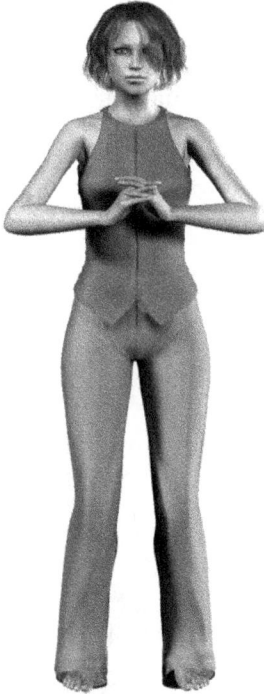

Slowly straighten up and
tuck in your backside.
Exhale gently as your
interlocked hands are at
the heart level

Inhale with your
interlocked fingers
facing your body.
Hold your breath
for a few moments
while you place
your hands on your
chest and let the
heat of the red light
warm your body.

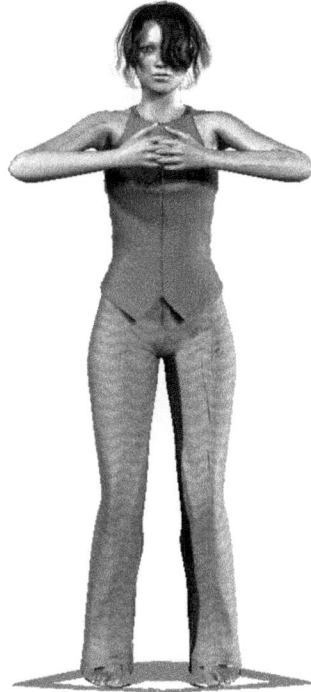

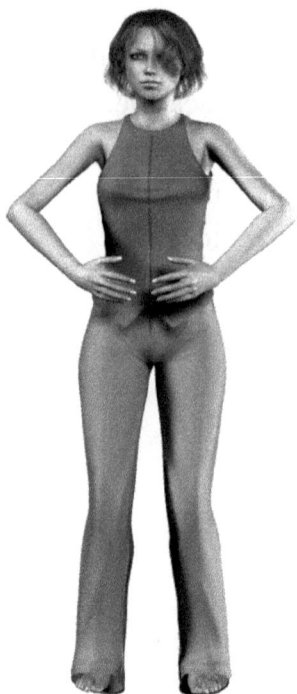

Let the hands come apart as you exhale and lower your hands to let them rest along your sides.

Keep breathing gently as you straighten your kness and relax into the standing posture.

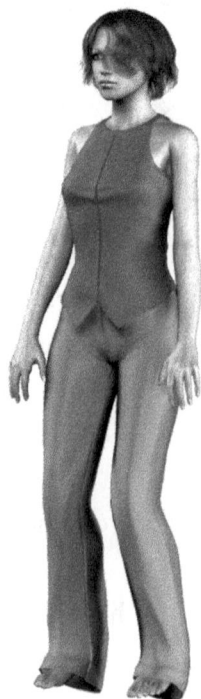

IV. Balancing the Air Element

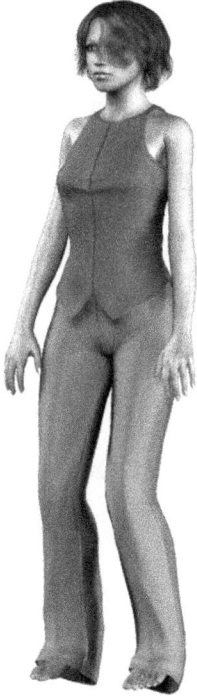

Stand with feet shoulder's width apart and hands by the sides. Relax your shoulders and tuck in the hips, aligning the back of the head with the tailbone.

Inhale and slowly raise your straight arms in front of your chest. While raising the arms, try to wriggel your fingers.

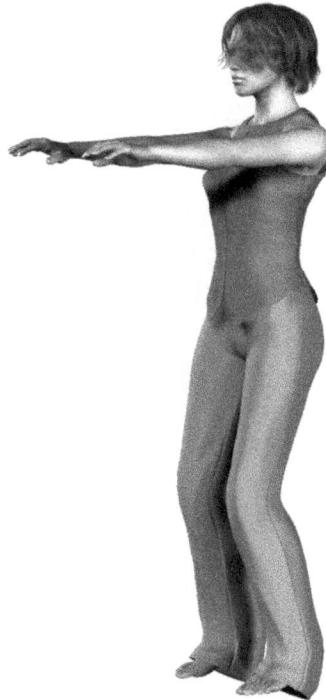

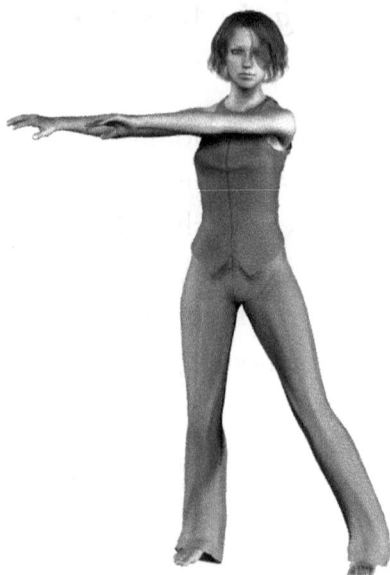

Exhale and swing your arms to the right. Shift your weight to the right leg. Then inhale and bring the arms back to the front.

As you exhale next, you swing your arms to the left, while shifting your weight to the left leg.
Inhale and swing the arms to the front. The weight is evenly distrib-uted between the legs.

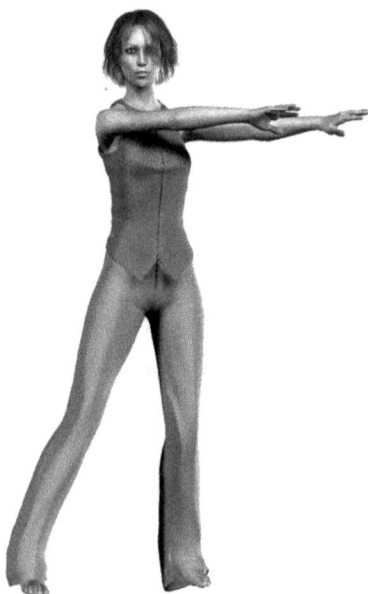

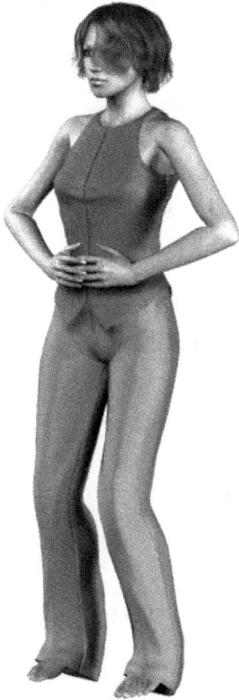

Exhale and bring the hands to the naval. Put both hands on the abdominal area. Imagine that you are absorbing the green light of the air element.

Remove your hands as you inhale and turn your hands downwards. Exhale and push the hands outward to the side. Tuck in your tailbone and straighten your knees. Relax with a few breaths.

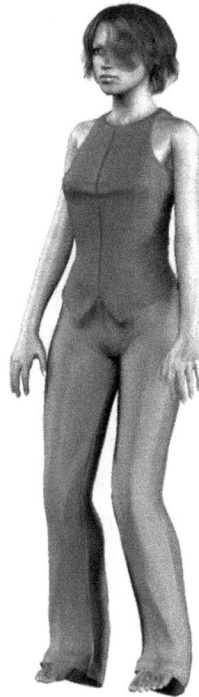

IV. Balancing the SpaceElement

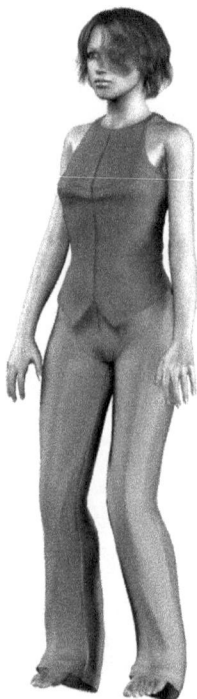

Stand with feet shoulder's width apart and hands by the sides. Relax your shoulders and tuck in the hips, aligning the back of the head with the tailbone.

Inhale and slowly raise the arms sideways and up to the forehead. The hands are then arranged in the symbol of the space element - the fingers steepled and touching to form a hollow structure. Visualize blue light in the hollow.

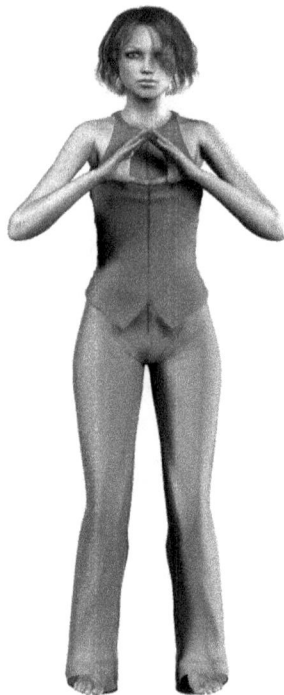

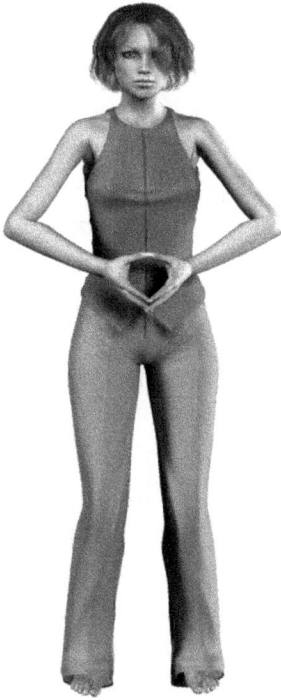

Exhale and bring the space
symbol from the chest
down to the naval area.
Then inhale and turn your
hands so that the touching
thumbs are uppermost.

Hold your breath for a few
moments as you absorb the
energy of space

Exhale and bring your
fingers apart, letting your
hands move to the sides.

Straighten your back and
kness. Relax and breathe
for a few minutes.

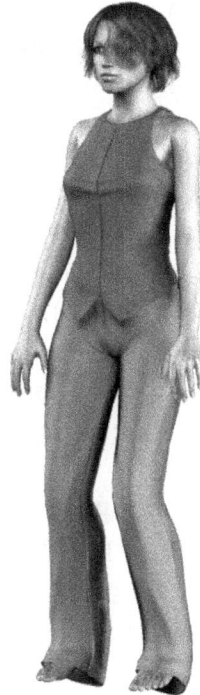

Conclusion

It has been my experience over a long period of time that the sytem of seven basic breathing techniques that I've introduced in this book has helped a diverse number of people with various health issues to attain improvements in their health and prospects of a longer life. This does not mean that they are a panacea for everything or that they can be relied on to cure all serious life-threatening diseases. This would of course be absurd. However, it is certainly possible to treat many otherwise difficult chronic conditions especially if they are stress related.

I've in various parts of the book alluded to the availability of scientific research that shows the therapeutic efficacy of the breath training techniques. However, I've not cited them specifically for two reasons: first, most of them are in journals or research papers that are not easily accessible to the general public and secondly, my vision for this as a practical workbook, rather than a rigorous text with citations that detract from that purpose. However, in this day and age, it is quite possible for those who wish to investigate further, to peruse and search the web for a lot of corroborating research.

Finally, it is my hope that you will not only read about it but practice the Prana Energy techniques and benefit from them. A word of caution is in order: a book is not a substitute for the guidance of a qualified teacher and so you must use common sense and care while doing these techniques.

May this program benefit you by improving your wellbeing, bring you peace of mind and an abundance of postive energy!

Books by Rudra Shivananda

Chakra selfHealing by the Power of Om

Yoga of Purification and Transformation

Surya Yoga - Healing by Solar Power

Breathe Like Your Life Depends On It

In Light of Kriya Yoga

Insight and Guidance for Spiritual Seekers

Practical Mantra Yoga for Self-Realization

Nada: The Yoga of Inner Sound

website: www.rudrashivananda.com
blog: www.sanatanamitra.com
www.youtube.com/user/KriyaNathYogi

About the Author

Rudra Shivananda, a disciple of the Himalayan GrandMaster Yogiraj Siddhanath, is dedicated to the service of humanity through the furthering of human awareness and spiritual evolution. He teaches that the only lasting way to bring happiness into one's life is by a consistent practice of awareness and transformation. He has developed healing programs utilizing the energy centers [Chakras] and Prana Energy techniques through breath.

Rudra Shivananda is committed to spreading the message of the immortal Being called Babaji. He teaches the message of World and Individual Peace through the practice of Kriya Yoga. As a student and teacher of yoga for more than 30 years, he is trained as an Acharya or Spiritual Preceptor in the Indian Nath Tradition, closely associated with the Siddha tradition. He lives in the San Francisco Bay area, and has given initiations and workshops in USA, Ireland, England, Japan, Spain, Brazil, Russia, Singapore, Malaysia, India, Australia, Canada and Estonia.

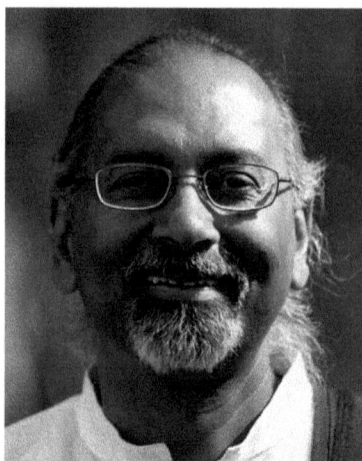